Eat What You Want!

Stop When You Want!

A No-Diet, Weight-Loss Program

Sora Vernikoff, M.A., M.S.

Green Mind Press

ISBN-13: 978-0692850237

ISBN-10: 0692850236

Book Disclaimer

The author and publisher disclaim all responsibility, liability, risk or loss (personal or otherwise) which might occur as a result of any use or misuse of any material in this book and will also have no responsibility for any adverse effects that arise directly or indirectly as a result of the material provided by this book. In addition, you should first consult your doctor or your other licensed health professional before starting any program in connection herewith.

This book was printed in the United States of America.

This book is dedicated to those people who want to make peace with food.

EAT WHAT YOU WANT!

STOP WHEN YOU WANT!

A No-Diet, Weight-Loss Program

Table of Contents

Part III-More Self-Stopping Information

Acknowledgements

There are so many people that I want to thank who helped make this book possible but first I want to begin by thanking God. It is my deep faith in a higher power that guided me and very generously supported me over the last two decades both in developing the work and in the writing of this book.

Then I want to thank all my clients that I've learned from. Yes, I developed The Program but it was you who gave it life by choosing to become a no-dieting, eat and stop yourself, make peace with food client.

Then I want to thank the endless number of people who read my book prior to publication. All of you know who you are! You all helped me write the very best teaching instructions possible and for that I am eternally grateful!

I also want to thank my parents for having me and I want to thank the gentle spirit of Karen Powell who was there for me at the very beginning of my no-dieting, self-healing journey *and who completely and whole-heartedly supported my vision!*

Then I want to thank David Rosenberg, my graphic design artist who stood by me and helped bring this book to completion through his great graphic design talents.

I also want to thank Jude Bijou, the author of Attitude Reconstruction *who gave me much wise, wise advice over the years.*

Then, I particularly want to thank, my digital assistant, Sarah Marshall. Not only is Sarah *an absolute digital wizard with the patience of an absolute saint* but she also supports the project in a very *meaningful* way.

And last, but by no means least, *I want to thank you the reader.* You, the reader who invested in this book because you believe in choice, the freedom that comes with having choice and the opportunity for unlimited possibilities that come with choice!

Thank you!

In Make Peace with Food,

Sora

My Story

Hi! My name is Sora Vernikoff and welcome to the land of self-stopping. Welcome to a program that will let you eat what you want, stop when you want and become forever thin and healthy all without having to diet. So before you learn why diets don't work and how to eat and stop yourself, I want to share my own weight loss story with you.

So for me it all started in kindergarten. My mom would always send me off to school in the morning with a bag filled with candy (I especially remember those pistachio nuts) and told me to have a good day. I also remember my breathing getting faster when my kindergarten teacher announced that it was Snack Time and passed around those wonderful chocolate chip cookies. Then back in college, I decided that I hated myself for having a "stomach" and for being less than "perfect". Along with my less than "perfect" decision came my commitment to tuna in water, extreme self-starvation and lots of bingeing behavior. Then about 10 years later after a series of dieting failures (where I'd lose the weight (felt great) and then would put it right back on) I decided that I didn't want to diet anymore. <u>I mean what was the point</u>? I did everything that the diet told me to do and yet I always regained the weight! Well, that was the day that I asked myself, "What's wrong with me? It can't be the diet, not the last word in weight loss or was it?" Now around this time, I also taught the toughest kids in East New York, Brooklyn. These were kids who walked, talked and threw chairs. However, after a while I learned to manage these kids really well and what truly puzzled me was that if food didn't walk or talk or throw chairs, why was it ruining my life and running my life?

Now, I must admit, that at the "same" time, I also had a roommate who served as a "thin" person role model. My roommate could have half a slice of rye bread and put the other half away or could have a few bites of a chocolate chip cookie and then throw the rest out. Well, I decided that I wanted those "same" choices. Why should she be able to eat and stop herself and I couldn't? So as a result of watching my classroom "management" techniques and my naturally "thin" roommate, *I had an idea…* That idea was "What would happen if I could vacuum out all the extra times a day that I thought about food?", "What else would I think about?" and "How would it change my life?" I simply wanted to stop dieting, *think less about food each day* and **let my weight permanently go.**

Well, that was the day that I stopped dieting and began journaling all of my daily eating experiences. I was simply determined to find out why I struggled so desperately with my food-thoughts and why I was so weight loss challenged.

So as a result of not dieting and journaling all of my daily eating experiences I reached my non-dieted twenty five pound weight-loss goal which I'm proud to say *that I've now kept off for over twenty years.*

Now at the "same" time that I reached my non-dieted weight loss goal, I also knew that I wanted to create a program that would help other fed up dieters be able to do the very same thing. As a result, I was able to transfer my classroom "management" techniques to food "management" techniques and Sora's Weight Loss "Management" Program was born.

Now I also want to add here "that Sora's Weight-Loss "Management" Program is not a nutritionally based weight loss program." Bookstore shelves are lined with nutritionally based weight loss programs and yet America's obesity rates have sky rocketed to epidemic proportion. Sora's Weight-Loss "Management" Program is a no diet, "food-thought" management program built around two specific types of behavior modification techniques. These two behavior modification techniques <u>only</u> teach you how to eat and stop yourself. Then *once you've learned how to eat and stop yourself,* you'll be making healthier food choices without any sense of deprivation *and you'll reach your non-dieted weight-loss goal.*

So why not stop dieting *and make peace with food today?*

I did it *and I know that you can too!*

In Make Peace with Food,

Sora

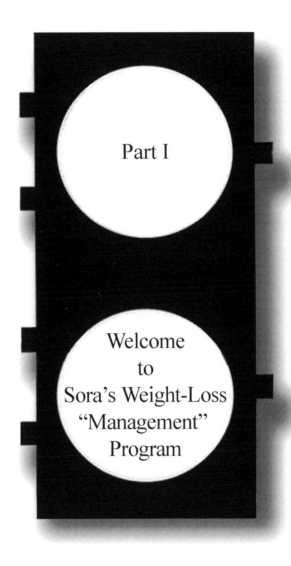

Part I

Welcome
to
Sora's Weight-Loss
"Management"
Program

Chapter 1

Why Don't Diets Work?

Before you learn how to use Sora's Weight-Loss "Management" Program (how to eat

what you want, stop when you want and become forever thin and healthy) it's important

to understand why diets don't work.

Diets don't work because a diet is a group of rules created by other people. These

other people tell you what to have, how much to have and even when to have what. In

addition, the diet tells you not to pay attention to your own food-thoughts. That it's

important to ignore your own food-thoughts because it's how you think about food that

brought you to this diet in the first place.

So now let's turn to the next page where you'll find Chart #1, also called Why Diets

Don't Work! This chart will help you understand how diets are set up and therefore why

they don't work.

Chart #1
Why Diets Don't Work!

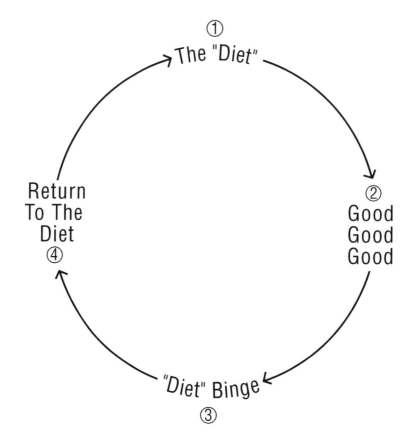

① The "Diet"

② Good Good Good

③ "Diet" Binge

④ Return To The Diet

So when you go on a diet (as shown at the #1) you've decided to follow the rules of "that" diet to lose your weight.

Now as you move around the circle to the #2 you'll see the term, Good, Good, Good. Good, Good, Good means that you've been following the rules of your diet and that you're losing your weight. But then as you continue around the circle you'll get to the #3 and see the term "Diet" Binge.

When you "Diet" Binge you've decided that it's time to escape the rules of your diet. Now, practically speaking, "Diet" Bingeing is the only thing that you can do to get that relief. However, after you've "Diet" Binged (and feel miserably out of control because you couldn't stop yourself) you get depressed and experience low self-esteem. At that point, you're probably thinking to yourself, "I want to be thin so much, but look what I just did! What is wrong with me?"

So what do you find yourself doing next?

As shown at the #4 you return to your diet. You return to your diet because after your last "Diet" Binge you feel that there is no way that you can get thin without this diet.

But, diets don't work!

Diets don't work because they're not your rules!

They're rules made up by "other" people.

It's only Sora's Weight-Loss "Management" Program that gives you the choice (unlike when dieting), to eat what you want, stop when you want and become forever thin and healthy.

Don't you think that it's time that those choices become *your* choices?

Chapter 2

Why Do You Have a Weight Problem?

So now that we've spoken about why diets don't work, let's talk about what really causes

your weight problem.

To help me explain this to you let's look below at Chart #2 also called Why Do You Have

A Weight Problem?

Chart #2
Why Do You Have A Weight Problem?

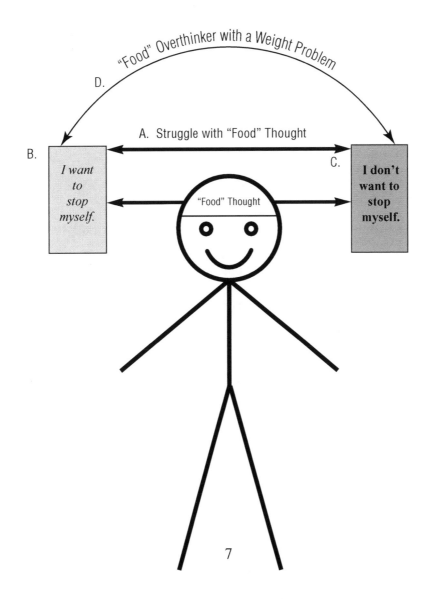

Looking at the letter A on this chart you'll see the phrase Struggle with "Food" Thought.

Struggle with "Food" Thought means that anytime that you think about "food" (see inside The Stick Figure's mind), that you don't know whether you're going to be able to stop thinking about "that" food or not.

So as shown in the light grey box to the left with the *italicized* print there will be times, when you think about "that" food that you feel that you can stop thinking about "that" food when you decide to and as a result you'll also feel that you can eat and stop yourself.

However, as shown in the dark grey box to the right with the **bold** print there will be other times, when you think about that "food" that you don't feel that you can stop thinking about "that" food when you decide to and as a result you also don't feel that you can eat and stop yourself.

As shown at the letter D, Sora's Weight-Loss "Management" Program says that because you never know whether you'll be able to stop thinking about each of your "food" thoughts when you decide to that you're what's called a "Food" Overthinker. That you're a person who thinks more about food in general than a person without a weight problem and as a result you feel stuck in one.

In Part II of this book, Learning How to Use The Program, you'll be learning how to eat and stop yourself whether as part of your Food-Thought Struggle (<u>your daily struggle</u>

with all of your "food" thoughts) you either want to stop thinking about the "food" that

you're thinking about or not.

Chapter 3

What are The Food Thoughts That You Can't Stop Thinking About?

Now Chart #3, Program "Food-Thoughts" shows you the two different types of food-thoughts that you might not be able to stop thinking about and which are causing your weight problem.

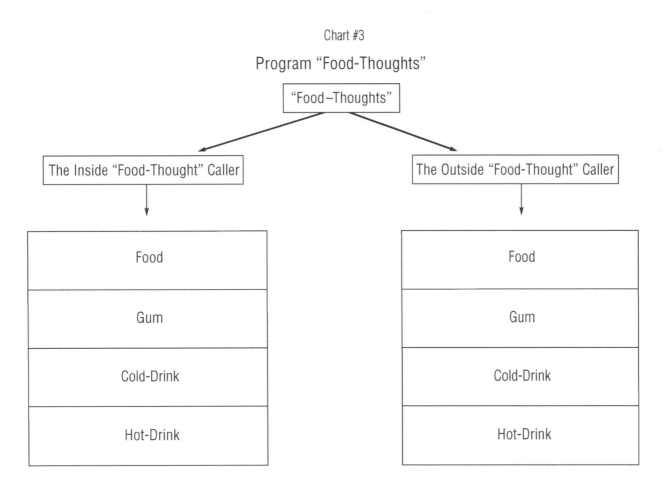

Chart #3

Program "Food-Thoughts"

On the top left of this chart, the first type of food-thought that you might not be able

to stop thinking about and which is causing your weight problem is called The Inside

"Food-Thought" Caller. To the top right of the chart, the second type of food-thought

that you might not be able to stop thinking about and which could also be causing your

weight problem is called The Outside "Food-Thought" Caller.

Now, an Inside "Food-Thought" Caller is any food that you first receive a signal for from

inside of your body. This signal might arrive as a sense of lightheadedness, as a sense of

growling in your stomach or as a sense of thirst. Once you receive any of these signals

then you'll think about what food your body might be calling for. Then, when you think

about a food that makes that signal feel better, that is the food that your body wants. That

is the food that whether you're eating or drinking which will make your body's inner

"hunger" or "thirst" signal feel better.

Now The Outside "Food-Thought" Caller unlike The Inside "Food-Thought" Caller

is any food or liquid that you decide to have but that you didn't first receive an inner

"hunger" or "thirst" signal for. They're the kinds of foods that you just "see" and want,

smell and want or just plain want.

So under the name The Inside "Food-Thought" Caller you'll see that there are 4 different

types of Inside "Food-Thought" Callers that you might receive a signal for.

If you receive an inner "hunger" signal then you're going to think about what "food" you want. If you receive an inner "mouth/discomfort" signal (to chew) but not on food then

you're going to think about what "gum" you want. If you receive an inner "cold-drink/

thirst" signal then you're going to think about what "cold-drink" you want and if you

receive an inner "hot-drink/thirst" signal then you're going to think about the "hot-drink"

that you want.

Now just as there are four different types of Inside "Food-Thought" Callers that you

might not be able to stop thinking about there are also four similar types of Outside

"Food-Thought" Callers that you also may not be able to stop thinking about. Those 4

similar types of Outside "Food-Thought" Callers are listed under the name The Outside

"Food-Thought" Caller and again they're food, gum, cold-drink and hot-drink.

Sora's Weight-Loss "Management" Program says:

> "That because you don't have the choice to stop thinking
>
> about any one of your "food" thoughts when you decide to
>
> or any combination of your food-thoughts when you decide
>
> to that you're food-thought challenged and as result, you
>
> feel stuck in a weight problem."

Well, you've just finished reading the first part of this book and you're ready to go to Part II, Learning How to Use The Program. It's here where you'll learn how to actually eat and stop yourself whether as part of your daily Food-Thought Struggle you either want to stop thinking about the "food" that you're thinking about or not. Then, after you've learned how to eat and stop yourself, you'll be able to comfortably reach your non-dieted weight loss goal in the shortest amount of time possible.

Sora

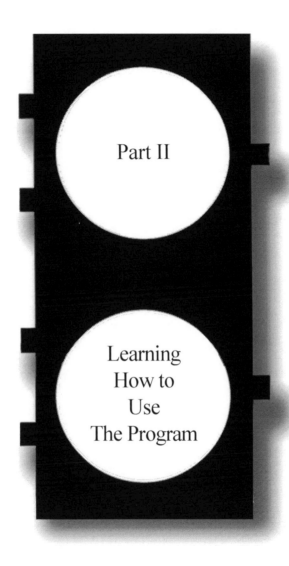

Part II

Learning
How to
Use
The Program

Chapter 4

How Can You "Eat" and Stop Yourself?

This chapter will teach you how to eat and stop yourself whether as part of your chewable "food-thought" struggle you either want to stop thinking about the "food" or "gum" that you're thinking about or not. I've included gum in this category since in Chapter 8 you'll be shown how gum can be used to decrease your weight loss "management" time.

Now to be able to eat and stop yourself, I'm going to first talk you through how to use The Stop-Chewable's Procedure and then you're going to have your own opportunity to practice.

So now let's turn to the next page where you'll find Chart #4, The Stop-Chewable's Procedure.

Chart #4

The Stop-Chewable's Procedure

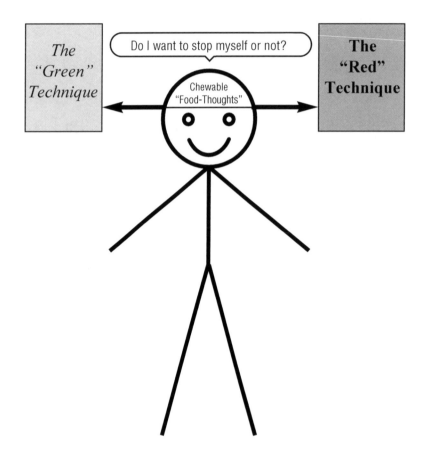

How Can You Eat and Stop Yourself by Using The Stop-Chewable's Procedure?

1. When using The Stop-Chewable's Procedure before you can have the food or gum that you're thinking about having you have to ask yourself the question:

"Do I want to stop myself or not?

(as shown above The Stick Figure's head)

2. Then you have to wait for your answer to arrive.

3. Then once your answer arrives you'll know whether you're going to have to use The "Green" Technique or The "Red" Technique to be able to eat and stop yourself.

Now if your answer arrives that you want to eat and stop yourself (that you want to stop thinking about the food or gum that you're thinking about) then you have to use The "Green" Technique (as shown in the light grey box to the left with the italicized print).

You'll get the food or gum that you want and ask yourself, "how much is enough?" and "how much is "too" much?" Then you have to actually set aside the amount that you decided was "too" much called your "Too" Much Marker. Then you can eat the amount that you decided was enough but never your "Too" Much Marker. This will let you know that you have eaten and stopped yourself.

Now if your answer arrives that you don't want to eat and stop yourself (that you don't want to stop thinking about the "food" or "gum" that you're thinking about) then as shown in the dark gray box to the right with the bold print you'll use The "Red" Technique.

You won't be able to have the "original" food or gum that you're thinking about having because you don't want to use a marker to be able to "eat" and stop yourself. Instead, you'll have to immediately switch your thinking from your "original" food

or gum thought to either your preselected "Binge" Food or your preselected "Binge" Gum. Once you've done that then by Technique definition you'll know that you can stop your "food" or "gum", Program "binge."

Now your preselected "Binge" Food which you'll soon be asked to select is the only food in this Program that you can "binge" on and know that you have stopped your Program food "binge." It should be a food that you really love that's between 180 and 280 calories. It must also be portable, easily available and not perishable. So a candy bar, a specific type of chip or a specific type of cookie would be your best bet.

In addition, once you pick your "Binge" Food you can never change it. Also, you can never eat it with a marker again simply because it's now your "own" special self-stopping "Binge" Food.

Now the guidelines for choosing your preselected "Binge" Gum are similar to the guidelines used when choosing your preselected "Binge" Food.

Your preselected "Binge" Gum which you'll also soon be asked to select is the only gum that you can "binge" on in this program and know that you have stopped your Program gum "binge." As when selecting your "Binge" Food it's very important that you choose a gum that you really like and that's easy to find. That's because as with your "Binge" Food, once selected, you can never change it or eat it with a marker again because it's now your "own" special, self-stopping "Binge" Gum.

So now let's get back to when you're using the actual technique.

Once your answer arrived that you didn't want to eat and stop yourself and you've immediately switched your thinking from your "original" food or gum thought to your preselected "Binge" Food or your preselected "Binge" Gum then you can go and get either one. Then in either case, you have to ask yourself, "How much is a comfortable amount to "binge" on?" You can then "binge" on that comfortable amount without having to first set aside your "Too" Much Marker and know that you have stopped either your Program food "binge" or your Program gum "binge."

So now it's your turn to practice. Turn to the next page!

So now you're going to practice how to use The Stop-Chewable's Procedure. First you'll

practice Program "eating" and then you'll practice Program "bingeing."   The instructions

are easy to follow. So have fun!

<u>The Stop-Chewable's Procedure Demo Form</u>

1. I decided to have some Cheese Bits.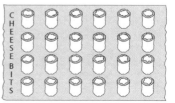

2. I'm focused to my Cheese Bits thought.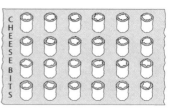

3. But before I buy it or have it, I have to ask myself:

"Do I want to stop myself or not?"

4. Then I have to wait for my answer to arrive.

5a. Pretend that your answer arrived that you wanted to

stop yourself. That means that you'll now use The "Green"

Technique.

l. So now pretend to pick up your Cheese Bits.

2. Now pretend to decide whether your Cheese Bits are

an Inside or Outside "Food" Caller. Do that now.

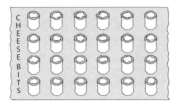

3. Then I will ask myself: How much is enough?

What is your answer?_____.

and

How much is "too" much?

What is your answer?_____.

4. Now pretend to tear off the amount which was "too" much

and pretend that you're setting it aside. Do that now.

5. I am now pretending to eat the amount that I decided was

enough but not my "Too" Much Marker. Do that now!

Well, congratulations! You've just successfully

finished practicing The "Green" Technique

with your Cheese Bits Caller. You

ate and stopped yourself because you set aside a

marker and had the amount that you decided was

enough.

I now want you to continue practicing this

procedure but only this time you're going to

practice using The "Red" Technique.

The Stop-Chewable's Procedure Demo Form

1. I decided to have some Cheese Bits.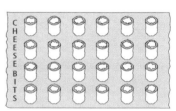

2. I'm focused to my Cheese Bits thought.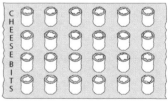

3. Then before I buy it or have it, I have to ask myself:

    "Do I want to stop myself or not?"

4. Then I have to wait for my answer to arrive.

5b. If my answer arrives that I don't want to

stop myself then I otherwise have to use

The "Red" Technique.

1. I WILL IMMEDIATELY SWITCH MY THINKING

FROM MY CHEESE BITS THOUGHT (TO STOP IT)

TO MY PRESELECTED "BINGE" FOOD, THE CANDY

BAR. 1 CANDY BAR

(Don't be concerned, at the end of this exercise

as previously mentioned you'll be able to select

your very own "Binge" Food.)

2. Then I will pretend to pick up The Candy Bar.

DO THAT NOW!

3. I WILL ASK MYSELF:

HOW MUCH OF THE CANDY BAR IS A

COMFORTABLE AMOUNT TO "BINGE"

ON?

WHAT IS YOUR ANSWER? _____.

4. Then after I've decided on that comfortable amount

I will "binge" on it.

5. <u>PRETEND TO DO THAT NOW. PRETEND TO</u>

<u>"BINGE" ON THAT COMFORTABLE AMOUNT</u>

<u>WITHOUT HAVING TO FIRST "SET ASIDE"</u>

<u>YOUR "TOO" MUCH MARKER.</u>

*So the only difference between this technique and The

"Green" Technique is that in this technique you can

only "binge" on your preselected "Binge" Food and you

don't have to first set aside a "chewable" management

marker.

Well, congratulations, again. You've just finished

practicing The "Red" Technique and were able

to stop your Cheese Bits thought even though

your original answer arrived that you didn't want

to. You were able to eat and stop yourself because

you "binged" on your preselected "Binge" Food,

The Candy Bar and that let you know that you

stopped your food "binge" behavior.

So now it's time for you to select your very own

"Binge" Food and pretend to write it in the box

below. When comfortable you can write it down

where you'll find it.

```
┌─────────────────────────┐
│                         │
│                         │
│                         │
│                         │
└─────────────────────────┘
```

And now that you've selected your very own

"Binge" Food you're ready to use this

procedure with any real food and be able to

stop yourself whether as part of your

"food" thought struggle you either want

to "eat" and stop yourself or not.

Well, now it's time to practice this procedure with gum. At this point, you're probably

thinking to yourself, "But, Sora, why do I have to use this procedure with gum when gum

is so low in calories?"

Program says, that part of your weight problem is that you don't have the choice to chew and stop yourself. This procedure lets you chew and stop yourself whether as part of

your "gum" thought struggle you either want to chew and stop yourself or not. Using this

procedure with your gum callers will also support you in shortening the amount of time

that it will take you to reach your non-dieted weight loss goal and again we'll talk more

about that in Chapter 8.

So just as you just did when practicing The Stop-Chewable's Procedure with food you're

going to do the same thing with gum. Have fun!

The Stop-Chewable's Procedure Demo Form

1. I decided to chew on some Gum Bits.

2. I'm focused to my Gum Bits thought.

3. But before I buy it or have it, I have to ask myself:

"Do I want to stop myself or not?"

4. Then I have to wait for my answer to arrive.

5b. *Pretend that your answer arrived that you wanted to*

stop yourself. That means that you will now use The

"Green" Technique.

1. So now pretend to pick up your Gum Bits.

2. Now pretend to decide whether your Gum Bits are an

Inside or Outside "Gum" Caller. Do that now.

```
G
U
M    [ ] [ ] [ ] [ ]
B    [ ] [ ] [ ] [ ]
I    [ ] [ ] [ ] [ ]
T    [ ] [ ] [ ] [ ]
S
```

3. Then I will ask myself: How much is enough?

What is your answer?_____ .

and

How much is "too" much? _____ .

4. Now pretend to tear off the amount which was "too" much

and pretend that you're setting it aside. Do that now!

5. I am now pretending to eat the amount that I decided was

enough but not my "Too" Much Marker. Do that now!

Well, congratulations again. You've just successfully

finished practicing The "Green" Technique

with your Gum Bits Caller-Teaching Aid. Again,

you were able to stop your "chewing" behavior

because you set aside a marker and had the amount

that you decided was enough.

As before, I want you to continue practicing this

procedure out-loud only this time you're going

to practice using The "Red" Technique.

The Stop-Chewable's Procedure Demo Form

1. I decided to chew on some Gum Bits.

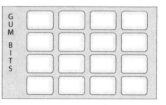

2. I'm focused to my Gum Bits thought.

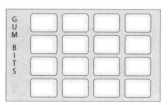

3. But before I buy or have it, I have to ask myself:

    "Do I want to stop myself or not?"

4. Then I have to wait for my answer to arrive.

5b. If my answer arrives that I don't want to stop

    myself then I otherwise have to use The

    "Red" Technique.

l. I WILL IMMEDIATELEY SWITCH MY THINKING

    FROM MY GUM BITS THOUGHT (TO STOP IT)

    TO MY PRESELECTED "BINGE" GUM, THE FUN GUM.

    FUN GUM

    (Don't be concerned, at the end of this exercise as

    previously mentioned you'll be asked to select

    your very own "Binge" Gum.)

2. Then I will pretend to pick up The Fun Gum.

    DO THAT NOW!

3. I WILL ASK MYSELF:

    HOW MUCH OF THE FUN GUM IS A COMFORTABLE

    AMOUNT TO "BINGE" ON?

    WHAT IS YOUR ANSWER? _____.

4. Then after I've decided on that comfortable amount

    I will "binge" on it.

5. <u>PRETEND TO DO THAT NOW</u>. <u>PRETEND TO</u>

    <u>BINGE" ON THAT COMFORTABLE AMOUNT</u>

    <u>WITHOUT HAVING TO FIRST SET ASIDE</u>

    <u>YOUR "TOO" MUCH MARKER</u>.

    *So the only difference between this technique and The

    "Green" Technique is that in this technique you can only

    "binge" on your preselected "Binge" Gum and you don't

    have to first set aside a "chewable" marker.

Well, congratulations, again! You've just finished

practicing The "Red" Technique and were

able to stop your Gum Bits thought even though

your original answer arrived that you didn't want

to. You were able to chew and stop yourself because

you "binged" on your preselected "Binge" Gum,

The Fun Gum and that let you know that you

stopped your gum "binge" behavior.

It's now time for you to select your very own

"Binge" Gum and pretend to write it in the box

below. Again, when you can, write it down

where you'll find it.

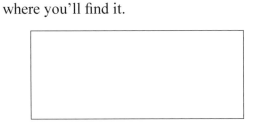

Now that you've selected your very own

"Binge" Gum you're ready to use this

procedure with any real gum and be able to

stop yourself whether as part of your

"gum" thought struggle you either want

to "chew" and stop yourself or not.

And now you're ready to use this procedure with your real food and real gum choices!

Make sure to always have your "Binge" Food and "Binge" Gum at hand (especially

your "Binge" Food) or you won't have the choice to eat and stop yourself if your answer

arrives that you don't want to stop yourself. Not having that choice will only take you

longer to reach your non-dieted weight loss goal.

Chapter 5

How Can You "Drink" and Stop and Yourself?

This chapter will teach you how to drink and stop yourself whether as part of your liquid "food-thought" struggle you either want to stop thinking about the cold-drink or the hot-drink that you're thinking about or not.

To do this you're going to learn how to use The Stop-Liquid's Procedure which is similar to The Stop-Chewable's Procedure.

Learning to use The Stop-Liquid's Procedure will help you shorten the amount of time that it will take you to reach your non-dieted weight loss goal and as with your Inside or Outside "Gum" Callers we'll talk more about that in Chapter 8.

So now, I'd like you to turn to the next page where you'll find Chart #5, The Stop-Liquid's Procedure.

Chart #5

The Stop-Liquid's Procedure

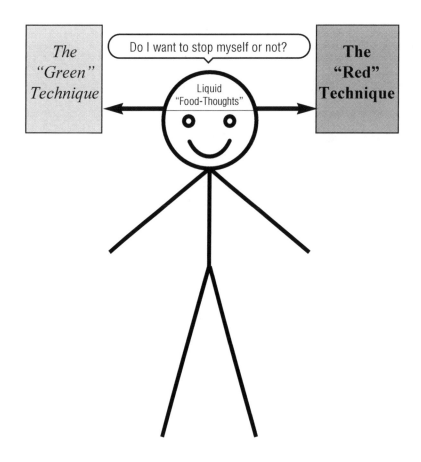

How Can You Drink and Stop Yourself by Using The Stop-Liquid's Procedure?

1. So as shown in Chart #5, similar to Chart #4 before you can have the cold-drink or hot-drink that you're thinking about having you have to ask yourself the question:

"Do I want to stop myself or not?

(as shown above The Stick Figure's head)

2. Then you have to wait for your answer to arrive.

3. Then once your answer arrives you'll know whether you're going to have to use either The "Green" Technique or The "Red" Technique to be able to drink and stop yourself.

Now if your answer arrives that you want to drink and stop yourself (that you want to stop thinking about the cold-drink or the hot-drink that you're thinking about) then you're going to use The "Green" Technique (as shown in the light gray box to the left with the italicized print).

You'll get the cold-drink or the hot-drink that you want and ask yourself, "how much is enough?" and "how much is "too" much?" Then you can drink the amount that you decided was enough remembering to leave over your "Too" Much Marker (the amount that you decided was "too" much). Then you have to glance at, or swish or shake your left over marker and that lets you know that you drank and stopped yourself.

Now if your answer arrives that you don't want to drink and stop yourself (that you don't want to stop thinking about the "cold-drink" or "hot-drink" that you're thinking about) then you'll use The "Red" Technique.

Again, you won't be able to have the "original" cold-drink or hot-drink that you're thinking about having because you don't want to drink and stop yourself by

remembering to leave over a "liquid" marker. Instead, you'll have to immediately switch your thinking from your "original" cold-drink or hot-drink thought to your preselected "Binge" Cold-Drink or your preselected "Binge" Hot-Drink. Once you've done that then by Technique definition you will know that you can stop your cold-drink or your hot-drink, Program "binge."

Now your preselected "Binge" Cold-Drink and your preselected "Binge" Hot-Drink are the only cold-drink and hot-drink that you can "binge" on in this Program and know that you have stopped your liquid "bingeing" behavior. So you're soon going to be asked to select a cold-drink and a hot-drink that are both easily available and that are either low in calories or non-caloric. You'll be asked to select two liquids that you really like because as with your preselected "Binge" Food and your preselected "Binge" Gum once chosen you can never change them. They're also both now your "own" special self-stopping "Binge" Liquids and you can never drink either of them with a marker again.

So now let's get back to when you're using the actual technique.

Once your answer arrived that you didn't want to drink and stop yourself and you've immediately switched your thinking from your "original" cold-drink or hot-drink thought to your preselected "Binge" Cold-Drink or your preselected "Binge" Hot-Drink, then you can go and get either one. Then in either case, you have to ask yourself, "How much is a comfortable amount to "binge" on?" You can then

"binge" on that comfortable amount without having to remember to leave over a "liquid" marker and know that you have stopped either your Program cold-drink "binge" or your Program hot-drink "binge."

So now it's your turn to practice. Turn to the next page!

So now you're going to practice how to use The Stop-Liquid's Procedure. First you'll practice Program "drinking" and then you'll practice Program "bingeing." The instructions as in the last chapter are easy to follow. So again, have fun with it!

The Stop-Liquid's Procedure Demo Form

1. I decided to have some juice.

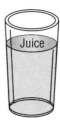

2. I'm focused to my juice thought.

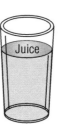

3. Then before I buy or have it, I have to ask myself:

"Do I want to stop myself or not?"

4. Then I have to wait for my answer to arrive.

5a. Pretend that your answer arrived that you wanted to

stop yourself. That means that you will now use

The "Green" Tecnique.

1. So now pretend to pick up your imaginery

paper juice glass.

2. Now pretend to decide whether your glass of

juice is an Inside or Outside "Cold-Drink" Caller.

Do that now.

3. Then I will ask myself: How much is enough?

    What is your answer?_____.

    and

    How much is "too" much?

    What is your answer? _____.

4. Now pretend to show yourself how much is enough

    and how much is "too" much by folding your

    imaginary paper juice glass.

5. Now pretend that you have drunk the amount of

    juice that you had decided was enough

    and then glance at your left over marker. Do that

now!

Well, congratulations! You've just successfully

finished practicing The "Green" Technique

with your Juice Caller. You drank enough

of your juice because you remembered

to leave over a marker and then you glanced at

it.

I now want you to continue practicing this

procedure but only this time you're going to

use The "Red" Technique.

The Stop-Liquid's Procedure Demo Form

1. I decided to have some juice.

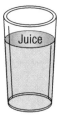

2. I'm focused to my juice thought.

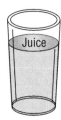

3. But before I buy it or have it, I have to ask myself:

Do I want to stop myself or not?

4. Then I have to wait for my answer to arrive.

5b. If my answer arrives that I don't want to

stop myself then I otherwise have to use

The "Red" Technique.

l. I WILL IMMEDIATELY SWITCH MY THINKING

FROM MY JUICE THOUGHT (TO STOP IT)

TO MY PRESELECTED "BINGE" COLD DRINK,

THE DIET SODA.

(Don't be concerned, at the end of this exercise as

previously mentioned you'll be asked to select

your very own "Binge" Cold-Drink.)

2. Then I will pretend to get The Diet Soda.

DO THAT NOW!

3. **I WILL ASK MYSELF:**

    HOW MUCH OF THE DIET SODA IS A

    COMFORTABLE AMOUNT TO "BINGE" ON?

    WHAT IS YOUR ANSWER? _____ .

4. **Then after I've decided on that comfortable amount I**

    will "binge" on it.

5. **PRETEND TO DO THAT NOW. PRETEND TO**

    "BINGE" ON THAT COMFORTABLE AMOUNT

    WITHOUT HAVING TO REMEMBER

    TO LEAVE OVER A "TOO" MUCH

    MARKER.

    *So the only difference between this technique and The

      "Green" Technique is that in this technique you can

      only "binge" on your preselected "Binge" Cold-Drink

      and you don't have to remember to leave over a marker.

    ***If you choose water as your "Binge" Cold-Drink then

      make sure to always use your same glass, same cup

      or same brand to "binge" from.

Well, congratulations again. You've just finished

practicing The "Green" Technique and were able

to stop your juice thought even though your answer

arrived that you didn't want to. You were able

to "drink" and stop yourself because you "binged"

on your preselected "Binge" Cold-Drink,

The Diet Soda and that let you know that you

stopped your cold-drink "binge" behavior.

Now, it's time for you to select your very own

"Binge" Cold-Drink and pretend to write it in the

box below. When you can, write it down

where you'll find it.

Now that you've selected your very own

"Binge" Cold-Drink you're ready to use this

procedure with any real cold-drink and be able

to stop yourself whether as part of your

"cold-drink" thought struggle you either

want to "drink" and stop yourself or not.

Well, now it's time to practice this same procedure with hot-drinks.

The Stop-Liquid's Procedure Demo Form

1. I decided to have some soup.

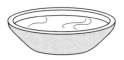

2. I'm focused to my soup thought.

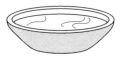

3. But before I buy it or have it, I have to ask myself:

Do I want to stop myself or not?

4. Then I have to wait for my answer to arrive.

5a. *Pretend that your answer arrived that you wanted*

to stop yourself. That means that you will now

use The "Green" Technique.

1. *So now pretend that you have your bowl of*

soup in front of you.

2. *Now pretend to decide whether your bowl*

of soup is an Inside or Outside "Hot-Drink"

Caller. Do that now.

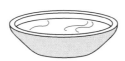

3. *Then I will ask myself: How much is enough?*

What is your answer? _____.

and

How much is "too" much?

*What is your answer?*_____.

4. *Now pretend to show yourself how much is enough*

and how much is "too" much by folding your

imaginary paper bowl of soup.

5. *Now pretend that you have drunk the amount of*

soup that you decided was enough and then glance

at your left over marker. Do that now!

Well, congratulations! You've just successfully

finished practicing The "Green" Technique

with your soup caller. You drank enough of your

soup because you remembered to leave over a

marker and then you glanced at it.

I now want you to continue practicing this

procedure but only this time you're going to

use The "Red" Technique.

The Stop-Liquid's Procedure Demo From

1. I decided to have some soup.
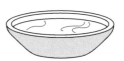

2. I'm focused to my soup thought.
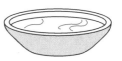

3. But before I buy or have it, I have to ask myself:

"Do I want to stop myself or not?"

4. Then I have to wait for my answer to arrive.

5b. If my answer arrives that I don't want to

stop myself then I have to otherwise use

The "Red" Technique.

I. I WILL IMMEDIATELY SWITCH MY THINKING

FROM MY SOUP THOUGHT (TO STOP IT)

TO MY PRESELECTED "BINGE" HOT-DRINK,

FUN TEA.

(Don't be concerned, at the end of this exercise

as previously mentioned you'll be able to

select your very own "Binge" Hot-Drink.)

2. Then I will pretend to get The Fun Tea.

DO THAT NOW!

3. I WILL ASK MYSELF:

HOW MUCH OF THE FUN TEA IS A

COMFORTABLE AMOUNT TO "BINGE" ON?

WHAT IS YOUR ANSWER? _____.

4. Then after I've decided on that comfortable amount
   I will "binge" on it.

5. <u>PRETEND TO DO THAT NOW. PRETEND TO
   "BINGE" ON THAT COMFORTABLE AMOUNT
   WITHOUT HAVING TO REMEMBER
   TO LEAVE OVER A "TOO" MUCH
   MARKER.</u>

   *So the only difference between this technique and The
   "Green" Technique is that in this technique you can only
   "binge" on your preselected "Binge" Hot-Drink and you
   don't have to remember to leave over a "liquid" marker.

Well, congratulations, again. You've just finished

practicing The "Red" Technique and were able to

stop your soup thought even though your original

answer arrived that you didn't want to. You were

able to stop yourself because you "binged" on your

preselected "Binge" Hot-Drink, Fun Tea and that let

you know that you stopped your hot-drink "binge" behavior.

52

Now it's time for you to select your very own

"Binge" Hot-Drink and pretend to write it in the

box below. Again, when you can, write it down

where you'll find it.

```
┌─────────────────────────────┐
│                             │
│                             │
│                             │
│                             │
└─────────────────────────────┘
```

Now that you've selected your very own "Binge"

Hot-Drink you're ready to use this procedure with

any real hot-drink and be able to stop yourself

whether as part of your "hot-drink" thought struggle

you either want to "drink" and stop yourself or not.

Well you've just learned how to drink and stop yourself and now you'll be able to have

any real cold-drink or any real hot-drink that you want and be able to stop yourself

whether as part of your liquid "food-thought" struggle you either want to drink and stop

yourself or not.

In addition, before we go on to the next chapter I just want to remind you of one very

important thing. When using The Stop-Liquid's Procedure similar to when using The

Stop-Chewable's Procedure always make sure to have your "Binge" Cold-Drink and

your "Binge" Hot-Drink "at" hand. Again, that's because if they're not "at" hand then

you won't have the choice to drink and stop yourself and it will only take you that much

longer to reach your non-dieted weight loss goal.

Chapter 6

How Can You "Bloat" and Stop Yourself?

You're now going to learn how to use The Bloatable's Procedure to be able to "bloat"

and stop yourself. Program tells you that when you "bloat" that you've decided to have

a low caloric type of food such as salad or soup for a stuffed stomach instead of having a

higher caloric type of food such as a candy bar for a non-stuffed stomach.

So let's talk about when you might decide to bloat yourself.

You've been running around all day doing errands and feel tired. You plan to drop

off your clothes at the dry cleaners, and then you're going to have dinner with friends.

However, to the right of the dry cleaners is your favorite doughnut shop and you see a

fabulous "pink" glazed doughnut in the window that you'd really like to have. So at

that moment, there's a part of you that would like to have that fabulous "pink" glazed

doughnut and then there's another part of you that would really like to save those calories

to have at dinner.

Well, about this time, you feel caught between a rock and a hard place.

However, Program tells you that in this kind of situation that you do have a choice

without experiencing any sense of deprivation. That you have the choice to either

Program "eat" the "pink" glazed doughnut with a marker or that you can otherwise bloat your stomach on a low caloric type of food such as salad or soup to be able to wait more comfortably for your dinner with friends.

So let's say for teaching purposes that you've decided that you'd rather bloat and save your calories for your dinner with friends.

It's making the choice to bloat, instead of having that fabulous "pink" glazed doughnut which is the first step (as shown on the next page) of The Bloatable's Procedure.

Chart #6

The Bloatable's Procedure

I'm thinking of having a "pink" glazed doughnut (a high caloric type of food) but because I want to use those calories to eat out tonight I've decided to "bloat" instead.

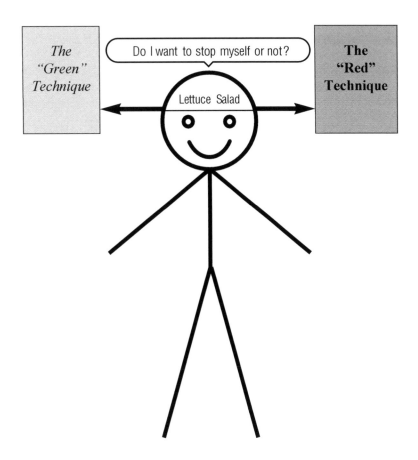

Now as soon as you've decided that you want to "bloat", you happen to see a Lettuce

Salad (see inside the Stick Figure's mind) in the deli window to the left of the dry cleaner

and you decide to "bloat" on The Lettuce Salad instead.

However, because The Lettuce Salad is a chewable (remember, you can also bloat on a

liquid) you also want the choice to "bloat" and stop yourself. So before you can have

The Lettuce Salad you have to ask yourself, "Do I want to stop myself or not?" and then you have to wait for your answer to arrive.

If your answer arrives that you want to bloat and stop yourself, then you'll use The "Green" Technique.

You'll get The Lettuce Salad that you want and ask yourself, "how much is enough?" At the same time that you're asking yourself, "how much is enough?" you'll also have to decide how much is "too" much. Then you'll have to actually set aside the amount that you decided was "too" much called your "Too" Much Marker. Then you can bloat "eat" the amount that you decided was enough, but never your "Too" Much Marker. This will let you know that you have bloat "eaten" and stopped yourself.

Now if instead, your answer arrives that you don't want to bloat and stop yourself but that you want to bloat and "binge" then you won't be able to use The "Green" Technique but you'll otherwise have to use The "Red" Technique.

Similar to when using The "Red" Technique in The Stop-Chewable's Procedure and similar to when using The "Red" Technique in The Stop-Liquid's Procedure you won't be able to have The Lettuce Salad that you're thinking about because you don't want to use a marker to bloat and stop yourself. Instead, you'll have to otherwise immediately switch your thinking from your Lettuce Salad thought to your preselected Bloat "Binge" Food. Once you've done that then by Technique

definition you'll know that you can stop your Program bloat "binge" behavior.

Now your preselected Bloat "Binge" Food, is the only "bloat" food that you can "binge" on and know that you have stopped your bloat "binge" behavior. You'll soon be asked to select a Bloat "Binge" Food which you have to make sure is not a seasonal fruit like honeydew or watermelon. You also have to make sure that it's the kind of "bloat" food that you really like and which is easy to find and portable. Also keep in mind that as with your four other preselected "Binge" Foods it's now your "own" special self-stopping Bloat "Binge" Food and you can never change it or bloat "eat" it with a marker again.

So now let's get back to when you're using the actual technique.

Once your answer arrived that you didn't want to bloat "eat" and stop yourself and you've immediately switched your thinking from your "original" Lettuce Salad thought to your preselected Bloat "Binge" Food then you can go and get it. Then you have to ask yourself, "How much is a comfortable amount to bloat "binge" on?" You can then bloat "binge" on that comfortable amount without having to first set aside a marker and know that you have stopped your bloat "binge" behavior.

So now it's your turn to practice. Turn to the next page!

So now you're going to practice how to use The Bloatable's Procedure. First you'll practice Program bloat "eating" and then you'll practice Program bloat "bingeing". The instructions are easy to follow. So have fun.

<u>Using The Bloatable's Procedure Demo Form</u>

1. I decided not to have the "pink" glazed

doughnut that I was thinking about.

2. I decided to "bloat" on a Lettuce Salad instead.

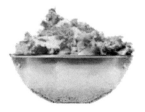

3. But before I buy it or have it, I have to ask myself:

"Do I want to stop myself or not?"

4. Then I have to wait for my answer to arrive.

5a. Pretend that your answer arrived that you wanted

to stop yourself. That means that you will now use

The "Green" Technique.

1. So pretend to get your Lettuce Salad.

2. Now pretend to decide whether your Lettuce Salad

is an Inside or Outside "Food" Caller. Do that

now.

3. Then I will ask myself:

How much is enough to "bloat" on?

What is your answer? _____ .

and

How much is "too" much?

What is your answer? _____ .

4. Now pretend to tear off the amount which was "too"

much and pretend that you're setting it aside. Do

that now.

5. I am now pretending to bloat "eat" the amount that I

decided was enough but not my "Too" Much Marker. Do

61

that now.

Well, congratulations! You've just successfully
finished practicing The "Green" Technique
with your Lettuce Salad Caller-Teaching Aid.
You bloat "ate" and stopped yourself because
you set aside a marker and had the amount that
you decided was enough.

I now want you to continue practicing this
procedure only this time you're going to
practice using The "Red" Technique.

Using The Bloatable's Procedure Demo Form

1. I decided not to have the "pink" glazed
doughnut that I was thinking about.

2. I decided to "bloat" on a Lettuce Salad instead.

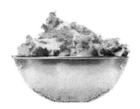

3. But before I buy it or have it, I have to ask myself:

   "Do I want to stop myself or not?"

4. Then I have to wait for my answer to arrive.

5b. If my answer arrives that I don't want to

stop myself then I otherwise have to use

The "Red" Technique.

l. I WILL IMMEDIATELY SWITCH MY THINKING

FROM MY LETTUCE SALAD THOUGHT

(TO STOP IT) TO MY PRESELECTED BLOAT

"BINGE" FOOD, THE RED APPLE.

(Don't be concerned, at the end of this exercise

as previously mentioned you'll be asked to

select your very own Bloat "Binge" Food.)

2. Then I will pretend to pick up The Red Apple.

   DO THAT NOW!

3. I WILL ASK MYSELF:

   HOW MUCH OF THE RED APPLE IS A

   COMFORTABLE AMOUNT TO BLOAT

   "BINGE" ON?

   WHAT IS YOUR ANSWER? _____.

4. Then after I've decided on that comfortable

   amount I will bloat "binge" on it.

5. <u>PRETEND TO DO THAT NOW. PRETEND TO</u>

   <u>BLOAT "BINGE" ON THAT COMFORTABLE</u>

   <u>AMOUNT WITHOUT HAVING HAD TO</u>

   <u>FIRST SET ASIDE A "TOO" MUCH</u>

   <u>MARKER.</u>

*So the only difference between this technique and

The "Green" Technique is that in this technique

you can only bloat "binge" on your preselected

Bloat "Binge" Food and you don't have to use a

marker.

***Also if you pick an apple as your Bloat "Binge" Food then it has to be the "same" type of apple all the time.

Well, congratulations again! You've just finished practicing The "Red" Technique and were able to stop your Lettuce Salad thought even though your original answer arrived that you didn't want to. You were able to bloat and stop yourself because you "binged" on your preselected Bloat "Binge" Food, The Red Apple and that let you know that you stopped your bloat "binge" behavior.

So now it's time for you to select your very own Bloat "Binge" Food and pretend to write it in the box below. Again, when you can, write it down where you'll find it.

So now that you've selected your very own

Bloat "Binge" Food, you're ready to use this

procedure with real bloatables whether as

part of your "bloatable" food thought struggle

you either want to "bloat" and stop yourself

or not.

Also keep in mind that you always have

to bloat "binge" on your "same" Bloat

"Binge" Food (in this case The Red Apple)

regardless of whether you want to

bloat "binge" on the "original" chewable

 or liquid bloatable that you were

thinking about having.

Important to remember!

Your 5 "Binge" Food Choices

Now is a good time to review your 5 "Binge" Food choices and to make sure to remind yourself to write them down somewhere when you can, so you can refer to your choices if you need to. Why don't you do that now!

My "Binge" Food is_____.

My "Binge" Gum is_____.

My "Binge" Cold-Drink is_____.

My "Binge" Hot-Drink is_____.

My Bloat "Binge" Food is_____.

Well, congratulations again! You've just learned how to eat and stop yourself, drink and stop yourself and bloat and stop yourself whether you wanted to stop thinking about the "food" thought that you were thinking about or not. You're now ready to go to Part III of this book, More Self-Stopping Information. Here you'll learn more information about how The Program works in supporting you in reaching your non-dieted weight loss goal.

Sora

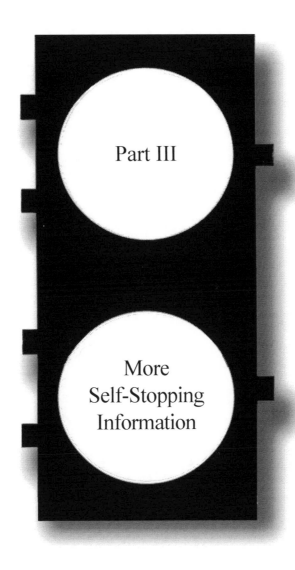

Part III

More
Self-Stopping
Information

Chapter 7

How Does Recording Help You Stop?

Below you'll find Chart #7, a copy of The Daily Program Form. This form can be

used on a daily basis to record your self-stopped "eating", "drinking" and "bingeing"

experiences. As you can see this form has been filled out to give you an idea of what

a filled out form might look like. However, there's a blank copy of the form in your

appendix which you can make copies of and use on a daily basis.

Chart #7
The Daily Program Form

Date: Jan. 1, 1991   Weight: 155 1/2

Sora's Weight-Loss "Management" Program		
Program "eat" ("Too" Much Marker)	**Program "drink"** ("Too" Much Marker)	**Program "binge"** (5 "Binge" Foods)

8:45 1 box 6 "Chocolate" 300
      mini donuts
	8:45 1 cup coffee 0	8:30 1 Mars Bar 240 384
		      "part of" another
		      Mars Bar 144

12:30 Turkey Sandwich 370
      on rye with 2T
      mustard
	10:30 1 cup coffee 0
	
	1:00 Diet Chocolate Soda 0
		3:10 3 Red Delicious
		      Apples 270

3:13 3 Oreos 150	4:00 Diet Chocolate Soda 0	

7:00 1 Shrimp Cocktail 100 166
      mixed green salad 48
      with mustard
      dressing 18		

10:37 3 packs sunflower 135 seeds		
Calories: 1121	Calories: 0	Calories: 654
Today's Caloric Intake: 1775		

© 1992 VERNIKOFF

So right now, you're probably thinking, "But Sora, why do I have to record my daily food choices?" Well, the reason why it's so helpful to record your daily food choices is to be able to *see* what you are doing. You'll be able to *see* if your weight is coming off as quickly as you'd like it to or whether you're having "too" many calories.

So when using this form, anytime you "eat" a chewable using a marker then record your "eating" experience in the first column called Program "eat" ("Too" Much Marker). Then anytime you "drink" a liquid using a marker, record your "drinking" experience in the second column called Program "drink" ("Too" Much Marker) and then anytime you "binge" on any of your "Binge" Foods then record your "bingeing" experience in the third column called Program "binge" (5 "Binge" Foods).

Think of your Daily Program Form as a computer print-out which shows you all of your daily self-stopped, "chewing" and "drinking" experiences.

Learn from it and have fun with it!

Chapter 8

What are Three Special Weight Loss "Management" Strategies?

Now let's talk about what you can do if you've been successfully using your markers

and your five "Binge" Foods but your weight isn't coming off as quickly as you'd like it

to. Here's the good news, The Program has three additional weight-loss "management"

strategies that can help move you along.

Strategy #1

Your first weight-loss "management" strategy as shown below in Chart #8a is called The

"Minimizer" Technique.

Chart #8a
The "Minimizer" Technique

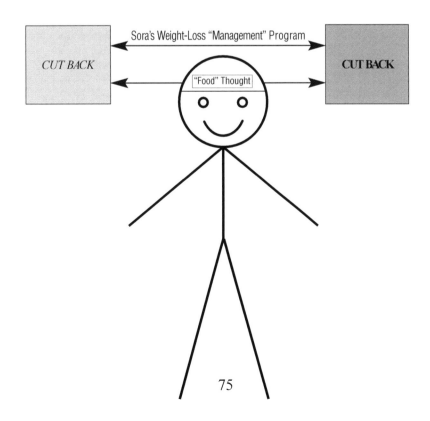

The "Minimizer" Technique tells you that if your weight isn't coming off as quickly as you'd like it to then just cut back when food "eating" with a marker or cut back when food "bingeing" on your "Binge" Food.

Strategy #2

Now if you've tried The "Minimizer" Technique and that's not working then look below at Chart #8b where you'll find The "4" Technique.

Chart #8b
The "4" Technique

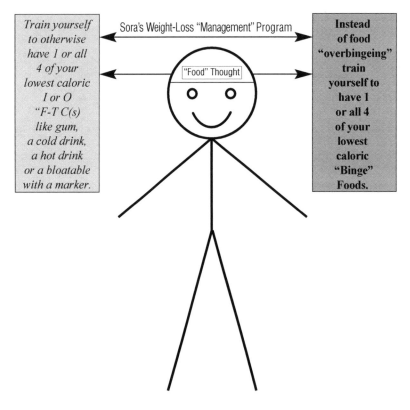

Train yourself to otherwise have 1 or all 4 of your lowest caloric I or O "F-T C(s) like gum, a cold drink, a hot drink or a bloatable with a marker.

Sora's Weight-Loss "Management" Program

"Food" Thought

Instead of food "overbingeing" train yourself to have 1 or all 4 of your lowest caloric "Binge" Foods.

The "4" Technique tells you that you have to train yourself to think differently now when you're about to have those "too" many calories.

The technique says (as shown by the *italicized* print in the light grey box to the left) that if you see that you're about to have "too" many calories when using a marker then you have the choice to have your 4 lower caloric foods with a marker instead. Those 4 lower caloric foods would be: gum, a cold-drink, a hot-drink or a bloatable.

However, The "4" Technique also says (as shown by the **bold** print in the dark grey box to the right) that if you're about to "overbinge" on your "Binge" Food then you also have the choice to have your 4 lower caloric "Binge" Foods instead. Your 4 lower caloric "Binge" Foods would be: your "Binge" Gum, your "Binge" Cold-Drink, your "Binge" Hot-Drink or your Bloat "Binge" Food.

So if you look on the next page you'll find another illustration of this technique using all of the book's paper food-teaching aids.

 So check it out!

The "4" Technique

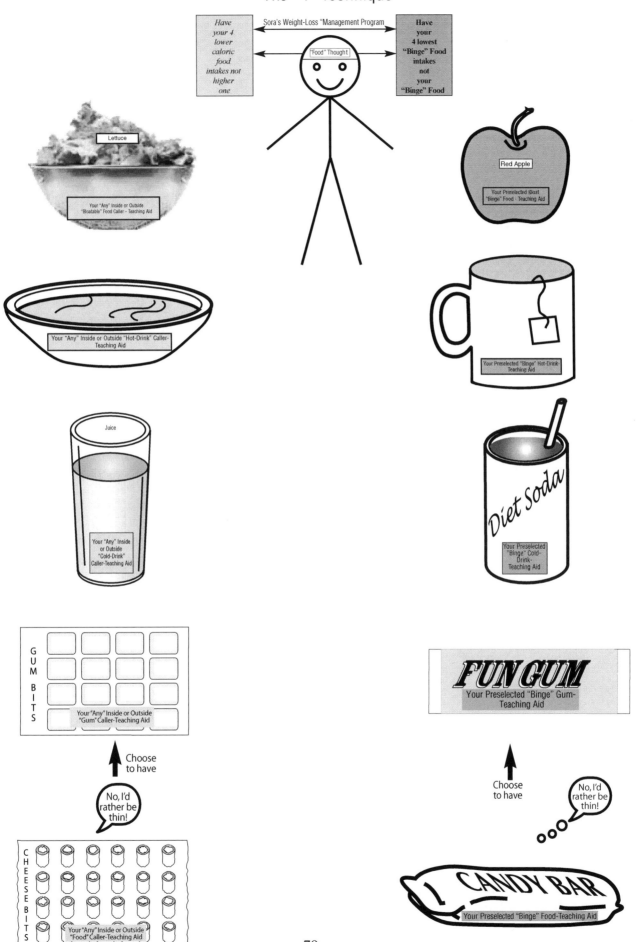

At this point, The Program says that if you've tried The "Minimizer" Technique and you've tried The "4" Technique and you're still struggling to reach your non-dieted weight loss goal then try Strategy #3, found below in Chart #8c which is called The "Boredom" Technique.

Strategy #3

Chart #8c
The "Boredom" Technique

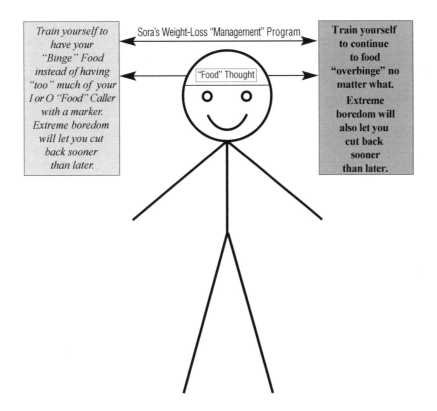

The "Boredom" Technique says (as shown in the light grey box with the *italicized* print to the left) that if you're about to food "overeat" then you should "binge" on your "Binge" Food instead. That otherwise bingeing on your "Binge" Food (instead of additionally food "overeating") will let you get bored more quickly with your extra "Binge" Food because you can never change it. The result of this is that it will make it easier for you to cut back sooner than later.

In addition, The "Boredom" Technique says (as shown by the **bold** print in the dark grey box to the right) that if you see that you're food "overbingeing" on your "Binge" Food (and that's keeping your weight on) then what you have to do is to train yourself to continue to food "overbinge" without going back to food "overeating". Again, because you can never change your "Binge" Food this will also make it easier for you to cut back in a shorter amount of time.

So if you look on the next page you'll find another illustration of this technique, again using the book's paper food-teaching aids.

So check it out!

The "Boredom" Technique

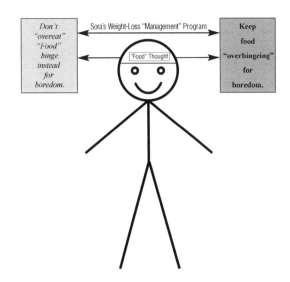

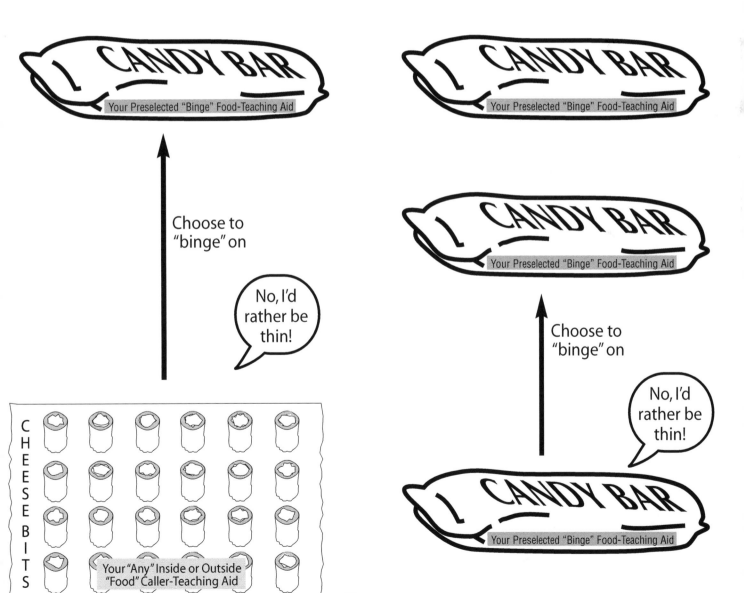

One additional thing that I'd like you to keep in mind is not to be afraid of food

"overbingeing." It's only by food "overbingeing" on your "Binge" Food that you'll

create the extreme kind of boredom with your "Binge" Food that is necessary for

you to make that comfortable choice to cut back. That is to cut back on your food

"overbingeing" without going back to food "overeating" with a marker. This technique

will let you reach your permanent non-dieted weight loss goal in the shortest amount of

time possible. So try it!

Chapter 9

Letters from Program Self-Stoppers

In this chapter I wanted to share some of the many notes and letters that I received from Program self-stoppers. I hope that you find them as inspiring to read as I have.

Dear Sora,

I had to write to say Thank You. I went to the doctor for the results of my physical on Thursday. My cholesterol is the lowest it has ever been, 131. My triglycerides were over 300 four weeks ago and now they were 132. I've lost 9 pounds and my stomach is half of what it was: pants are looser and I feel great. My energy level for playing tennis, is improving and I ride my stationary bike at a faster speed.

All I do is ask myself if I can stop. I take home half a meal when I dine out, which makes for a great meal the next night. I can't seem to finish a bag of popcorn any more which is amazing and without feeling any deprivation, I've been able to cut back on my favorite pretzels.

So…THANK YOU…

I feel better both physically and emotionally.

S.K.

Putnam Valley, New York

Dear Sora,

Thank you, thank you, thank you. After all these years, I have finally found a way to eat

what I want and lose weight at the same time.

After listening to you and practicing your program, I realized that all these years I have

been attempting to maintain diets by depriving myself of the foods I loved.

With your program not only can I eat what I want and stop when I want, I can even have

my favorite "binge foods."

Who would have thought that by just planning the portion size and leaving markers that

I would find the perfect lifetime plan. More importantly, I would succeed in losing and

maintaining the weight without ever feeling deprived!

Thanks again for all your personal imput and I wish you continued success.

M.S.

Edgewater, New Jersey

Dear Sora,

I just wanted to write to tell you how pleased I am with your Weight-Loss "Management" Program. The name of your program says it all…because for the first time in years, I'm actually able to "manage" my weight-loss, rather than be "managed" by someone else's idea of a diet that's unrealistic and impossible to follow.

You made me realize that dieting is only a temporary fix. I guess I should have known that because whenever I would go "on" a diet, I'd lose weight, only to gain it back when I went "off" the diet. Your program is one that I can follow for a lifetime, without fear of my weight constantly going up and down and then back up. I can finally give away all of those "fat clothes" of mine!

The best part is, I don't feel deprived. If anyone had told me that I'd be able to lose weight, and more importantly, keep it off, while still enjoying all of my favorite foods and snacks, I never would have believed it. I can't tell you how good it feels to be able to control what I eat, instead of being controlled by what I can't eat.

Thank you again for sharing your program with me.

J.M.

Fort Lee, New Jersey

Dear Sora,

Being in your weight loss program has helped me to cope with my weight problem, and I am more in tune to my body than ever before.

I also know when enough is enough which is very important to my daily intake.

Thanks to you I am taking more of an interest in my body.

I am forever grateful.

M.D.

Buford, Georgia

Dear Sora,

I have tried your plan and it really is manageable. I've lost 10 pounds in two months' time and have kept the weight off. I want to lose more weight and feel like I need a lot of structure, but I am able to apply Sora's ideas to my weight-loss choices and not feel so limited. Having "safety" foods has been a life-saver! Sora put her heart into this plan and it shows…she's thought of everything.

N.J.

New York, New York

Dear Sora,

I want to thank you for introducing and explaining to me your weight-loss "management" program. It is very effective and it is different from the other weight loss programs in that you can still have your favorite foods but you have the choice when to stop. You can eat what you like and still lose weight. It is an effective and interesting program and I really love the freedom to have any food that I want.

L.M.

New York, New York

Dear Sora,

Enjoyable program and different from other types of weight-loss classes.

The opportunity is there to "binge" on your favorite products in a way to avoid overeating.

I find that I'm better able to control my appetite and that in and of itself allows my weight-loss to remain steady.

Thanks for The Program.

P.S.

Brooklyn, New York

Dear Sora,

I love your fabulous self-stopping non-dieting program. I think that you're also a great teacher.

You made everything so easy. I love the markers. They help me not eat everything in sight. I will be using them the rest of my life. I've lost 10 pounds, feel confident about keeping them off and look forward to losing more weight.

Best Regards.

N.K.

Edgewater, New Jersey

Chapter 10

What are Some Self-Stopping Program Questions?

Now here are some popular program questions asked by my clients as well as by my seminar participants. See if they help you answer some of your questions about The Program as well.

Questions about The Stop-Chewable's Procedure and The "Green" Technique

1. If I don't use The Stop-Chewable's Procedure (which includes The "Green" Technique) can I become bored enough with my extra "food" thoughts to be able to choose a permanent non-dieted weight loss?

No, you can't. Right now, you don't have the choice to always be able to eat and stop yourself which leaves you thinking more a day about food than a person without a weight problem. Using The Stop-Chewable's Procedure which includes The "Green" Technique will give you the choice to eat and stop yourself. It's having this choice which will let you get bored with your extra "food" thoughts and let you reach your non-dieted weight loss goal. Can you realistically do this without The Stop-Chewable's Procedure and The "Green" Technique? The answer is no.

2. When my answer arrives that I want to stop myself, can I trust my answer?

Yes, always trust your answer, if it arrives that you want to stop yourself. It's the next step that you'll take to reach your non-dieted weight loss goal.

3. Why do I always have to first set aside a chewable "Too" Much Marker?

You always have to first set aside a chewable "Too" Much Marker before you "eat"

to see how much of the food that you want is enough. Once you "see" (by

setting aside a marker) how much of the food that you want is enough then you'll

know that you can eat and stop yourself.

4. What should I do with my chewable "Too" Much Marker?

If your chewable "Too" Much Marker is small then you're probably going to want to

throw it out. If it's large, then you might want to put it away and have it at another

time with a new chewable "Too" Much Marker.

5. What if I've Program "eaten" and still want more of the "same" food?

If you've just Program "eaten" and still want more of the "same" food then

you have to ask yourself, "Will having more of the "same" food help me to reach

my non-dieted weight-loss goal?" If you do decide that you do want "more" of the

"same" food then make sure to use your "original" "Too" Much Marker or set aside

a new one.

6. What if I use The "Green" Technique and I have "too" much?

If enough becomes "too" much then why not try one of your three special weight loss

"management" strategies as found in Chapter 8.

7. If I have a salad or full meal where there are a couple of ingredients do I have to first set aside a chewable "Too" Much Marker for "each" of the ingredients or for "each part "of" the meal"?

The answer to this question is yes. If you don't set aside a chewable "Too" Much Marker for "each ingredient "of" the salad" or for "each part "of" the meal" then you won't know how much of "each part "of" the salad" or how much "each part "of" the meal" is enough and then you won't have the choice to eat and stop yourself.

Questions about The Stop-Liquid's Procedure and The "Green" Technique

1. If I don't use The Stop-Liquid's Procedure (which includes The "Green" Technique) can I become bored enough with my extra "liquid" food-thoughts to be able to support a non-dieted weight loss?

Even though your "liquid" food-thoughts are probably lower in calories than your "chewable" food-thoughts it's also very important to have the choice to drink and stop yourself. That is to drink and stop yourself whether as part of your liquid "food-thought" struggle you either want to drink and stop yourself or not. So, the more you use The Stop-Liquid's Procedure (which includes The "Green" Technique) the more bored you will become with your extra "liquid" food-thoughts and yes, the easier it will become to support your non-dieted weight loss.

2. When my answer arrives that I want to stop myself, can I trust my answer?

95

Yes, as when using The Stop-Chewable's Procedure when your answer arrives that you want to stop yourself, then trust it. It's also the next step that you'll take to reach your non-dieted weight loss goal.

3. When using The "Green" Technique do I always have to leave over a liquid "Too" Much Marker?

Yes, when using The "Green" Technique you always have to remember to leave over a liquid "Too" Much Marker. Without leaving over a liquid "Too" Much Marker nothing you will have drunk will have been enough. This will only take you that much longer to reach your non-dieted weight loss goal.

4. What should I do with my liquid, "Too" Much Marker?

If your liquid "Too" Much Marker is small then you're probably going to want to throw it out. If it's large then you might want to put it away and then have it later with a new liquid "Too" Much Marker.

5. What if I've used The "Green" Technique with a liquid and still want more?

If you've used The "Green" Technique with your cold-drink or hot-drink and you still want more then make sure that you have enough in the can or glass to leave over another liquid "Too" Much Marker. If you don't have enough in your first glass or can to leave over a second liquid marker *then make sure to refill your glass or get a second can.*

6. What if I use The "Green" Technique and drink "too" much?

If enough of any liquid becomes "too" much and it's calorically affecting you reaching

your non-dieted weight loss goal then why not try one or all three of your weight-

loss "management" strategies as found in Chapter 8.

7. Can I use The "Green" Technique with wine, beer or alcohol?

All three of these are cold-drink liquids, so if your answer arrives that you want to

stop yourself, then why not?

Questions about The Bloatable's Procedure

1. Do I have to use The Bloatable's Procedure to manage my bloatables?

Again, if you don't use The Bloatable's Procedure to manage your bloatables (to

be able to "bloat" and stop yourself) then it will only take you that much longer to

reach your non-dieted weight loss goal.

2. When I ask myself, "Do I want to stop myself or not?" will an answer always arrive?

As when using The Stop-Chewable's Procedure and The Stop-Liquid's Procedure,

yes, your answer will always arrive. Always trust your answer. It's the next step

for you to take to reach your non-dieted weight loss goal.

3. What if I've used The "Green" Technique with a chewable bloatable and still want more?

If you've used The "Green" Technique with a chewable bloatable and still want more then make sure that you use your "original" chewable "Too" Much Marker or first set aside a new one.

4. What if I've used The "Green" Technique with a liquid bloatable and still want more?

If you've used The "Green" Technique with a liquid bloatable and still want more then make sure that you use your original liquid "Too" Much Marker or remember to leave over a new one.

5. Even though I dislike that "stuffed" feeling, do I have to "bloat"?

Bloating helps you wait more comfortably for your next higher caloric intake. That stuffed feeling is the trade-off for not otherwise having your higher caloric intake. If you think of that "stuffed" feeling as helping you to reach your non-dieted weight loss goal in a shorter amount of time then you might think of it differently.

6. How many times a day should I "bloat"?

You should bloat as many times a day as it feels comfortable.

7. Can I lose my weight without "bloating"?

Yes, you can lose your weight without bloating but it will only take you that much longer to do.

Questions about The "Red" Technique and Your 5 "Binge" Foods

1. If I "binge" on my "Binge" Food a lot, will I be eating healthy?

You might find yourself Program "bingeing" more than Program "eating" when you first start The Program because now you have the freedom to food "binge" and stop yourself. However, because you can never change your "Binge" Food you'll quickly get bored of it. This "boredom" will get you food "eating" more with a marker and in time your food choices will become more in tune with your body's inner "hunger" signals.

2. Won't I probably have more calories when I Program "binge" than when I Program "eat"?

No, just the opposite is true. Since you can never change your "Binge" Food it will get more boring to have (in less time) then the different foods that you can Program "eat" with a marker. So the answer to this question is no.

3. Can I ever use a chewable or liquid "Too" Much Marker with any of my 5 "Binge" Foods?

You can NEVER use a "Too" Much Marker with any of your five "Binge" Foods. Once a "Binge" Food only a "Binge" Food. Your five "Binge" Foods are now your five "own" special self-stopping "Binge" Foods and you can NEVER have any of them with a marker again.

4. Can I choose a multi-color or multi-flavor "Binge" Food or "Binge" Gum such as Jelly Beans or Fruit Chiclets?

The answer to this question is no. Choosing a multi-color, multi-flavor "Binge" Food or "Binge" Gum will only take you that much longer to get bored of and therefore it will only take you that much longer to reach your non-dieted weight loss goal.

5. Why can't I choose carrots as my "Binge" Food?

If you make carrots your "Binge" Food then you'd be on a diet and why would you want to do that?

6. Can I ever change any of my 5 "Binge" Foods?

No! No! No!

Once you've selected your "Binge" Food, your "Binge" Gum, your "Binge" Cold-Drink, your "Binge" Hot-Drink and your Bloat "Binge" Food you may never change any of them. You may never change any of them to make each of them as boring as possible in the shortest amount of time possible to help you reach your non-dieted weight-loss goal.

7. Why is it so important to have my 5 "Binge" Foods "at" hand?

If you don't have your 5 "Binge" Foods immediately available (that means "at" hand) and you want to "binge" then you won't know how much is enough and won't be able to stop yourself.

8. What would happen if I changed any one of my 5 "Binge" Foods?

If you change any one of your 5 "Binge" Foods then it will only take you that much longer to get bored with your extra food-thoughts and therefore reach your non-dieted weight loss goal.

Chapter 11

What are Some General Program User Questions?

Here are some general types of questions asked by my clients and I hope that they help you answer some of your general questions as well.

1. "Sora, I don't think a lot about food each day and yet I still have a weight problem. Why is that?"

   By Program definition if you feel that you have a weight problem then you do think more about food a day than a person without a weight problem. However, if you don't think that you think "too" much about food a day that's because you don't own your "extra" food-thoughts. Commitment to The Program will give you the choice to own your "extra" food-thoughts and that will give you the choice to let them go.

2. "Sora, why are my markers and my "Binge" Foods so important?"

   Your markers and your "Binge" Foods are your Food-Thought "Boredom" Patrol. They help you stop your food-thoughts and as a result make your extra food-thoughts and your extra "Binge" Foods extremely boring. When that happens, your weight will come off.

3. "Sora, I have a low metabolism. Will this Program still work for me?"

   Whether your metabolism is low or high you still want the choice to eat and stop yourself. If you have a low metabolism then you can adjust your food choices but

you still want the choice to eat and stop yourself.

4. "Sora, I don't chew gum. Do I have to?"

There's no law that says that you have to chew gum. But if you decide not to carry

around gum then The Program suggests that you carry around a small type of

"sucking" candy. This will support you during those more difficult times of your

day.

5. "Sora, do calories count?"

Yes, there is no denying that ultimately it's your daily average caloric intake which

will keep your weight off. However, using The Program gives you the choice not to

diet and become bored with your "extra" food-thoughts to become permanently

thin and healthy.

6. "Sora, should I buy a calorie book?"

It can't hurt. It can only help. After all, "Knowledge is power."

7. "Sora, will this Program let me make low fat, nutritional and healthy choices?"

Yes, you can have any food that you want in Program. If you want low fat and

nutritional foods then of course you can have them. However, what's important

to keep in mind is that it's not the low fat foods or the nutritional foods that will take

your weight off or more importantly keep it off. That what will take your weight off and keep your weight off is having the choice to always be able to eat and stop yourself no matter what type of foods you choose to have. Program gives you that choice.

8. "Sora, will this Program let me reconnect with my body's self-regulatory inner "hunger" and "thirst" signals?"

Yes, it definitely will. Once you get used to The Program and know that you are always able to eat and stop yourself, then you'll be able to wait comfortably for longer periods of time before you want to eat again. Having this ability to wait longer periods of time to eat will let you develop the patience to learn to listen for your own special inner "hunger" and "thirst" signals. Once you learn to do that then you'll be able to fill those signals with the food that your body wants in addition to knowing that you can stop yourself.

9. "Sora, will this Program take care of my cravings?"

When someone asks me if this Program will take care of their "cravings", I often feel that they attach a mystical quality to that word. The word craving as Program defined is a "food" thought whether it appears as an Inside or Outside "Food"-Thought Caller. In Program, you can have any food you crave but now you'll always have the choice to stop yourself. How great is that!

10. "Sora, I feel guilty when I Program "binge", even though I've been losing weight. Why is that?"

The reason that you might feel guilty when you Program "binge" is because every diet program tries to protect you from the part of yourself that doesn't want to stay on the diet and wants to "binge". However, when Program "bingeing" unlike when diet "bingeing" you always but always have the choice to stop yourself. Knowing that you can "binge" and stop yourself will let you reach your non-dieted weight loss goal in the shortest amount of time possible and so Program's motto is: "Binge to win and get forever thin."

11. "Sora, how long will it take me to reach my non-dieted weight loss goal?"

It will take you as long as it takes you to reach your non-dieted weight loss goal. Simply keep using your "Too" Much Markers, your five "Binge" Foods and when tempted to have "too" much of either always ask yourself, "What do I want more?, the extra calories or my weight-loss?" Then trust yourself because your answer will always arrive.

12. "Sora, does this Program guarantee weight-loss?"

This Program makes no guarantees. The only guarantee that The Program does make is that if you commit to The Program, <u>stay</u> committed to The Program, use your "Too" Much Markers and your five "Binge" Foods then a permanent non-dieted weight-loss is there for you to own.

13. "Sora, how many meals and snacks can I have a day in your Program?"

You can have as many meals and snacks as you want a day in this program.

However, it's important to see how your daily choices affect your non-dieted weight-loss goal.

14. "Sora, what time of the day can I have food?"

    When using this Program you can have any food any time of the day that you want.

15. "Sora, do I have to use a scale or The Daily "Recording" Form?"

    I think of the scale and The Daily "Recording" Form in the "same" way as I do the calorie guide. If it feels comfortable then use it. If it doesn't, then don't.

16. "Sora, isn't it my emotions which are causing my weight problem?"

    Your emotions <u>don't</u> cause your weight problem <u>but are aggravated by it.</u>
    What causes your weight problem is that you think more about food a day
    than a person without a weight problem and you don't always have the choice
    to eat and stop yourself. Once you learn how to use The Program and manage your
    "own" food-thoughts you'll have more time and energy to work on any other
    unresolved emotional issues. That's because you won't have all of those extra food-
    thoughts getting in your way.

17. "Sora, is exercise part of The Program?"

    Exercise is not a part of The Program. However, if exercising feels comfortable
    then do it. I strongly recommend it.

18. "Sora, what happens if one day I forget to use my markers or my "Binge" Foods?

If for whatever reason you don't use markers or your "Binge" Foods on any given

day then just pick yourself up and dust yourself off and go back to your self-

stopping management the next day.

19. "Sora, what's the best way to describe this Program to a friend?"

The best way to describe this Program to a friend is to keep it simple. Just tell your

friend that it's a non-dieting weight-loss program, that lets you eat what you want,

stop when you want and become forever thin and healthy.

20. "Sora, how can this Program help me at holiday parties or when eating out?"

Having your five "Binge" Foods available at holiday parties or when eating out will

make all the difference. If necessary, bring your "Binge" Food or "Binge" Gum

whenever you can. <u>Your "Binge" Foods will always act as your safety net.</u>

21. "Sora, what will I do if I travel, don't pack enough of my "Binge" Foods and find

myself without them?"

If you find yourself in a city, state or country without your "Binge" Foods then just

look for the same type of food(s) in the same color packaging. This will let you

keep the same type of self-stopping relationship that you had with your original

"Binge" Food(s) as best as possible.

22. "Sora, many members of my family are overweight. Isn't it possible that it's a fat

gene that is causing my weight problem?"

Today scientists are working to show you that there's a fat gene and that people with that fat gene lean towards being overweight. However, whether there is a fat gene or not, Program says that as a person with a weight problem that you are food-thought challenged. That you think more about food a day then a person without a weight problem and that's why you have a weight problem. That it's only by learning how to eat and stop yourself (to manage your "own" food-thoughts) that you can get bored enough with your extra food-thoughts to make the choice to become forever thin and healthy.

23. "Sora, I enjoy having wine, beer or alcohol. How can I manage that?"

If you drink wine, beer or alcohol then you'll manage it the same way that you'd manage any cold-drink. Before you drink it, you'll ask yourself, "Do I want to stop myself or not?" and then you'll use one of The Stop-Liquid's Procedure's two self-stopping techniques to be able to drink and stop yourself. <u>However, if you drink a lot of wine each week or a lot of beer each week or for that matter a lot of alcohol each week then you should select your very "own" special, self-stopping Wine "Binge" Food, Beer "Binge" Food or Liqueur "Binge" Food.</u> Doing this will let you make sure that you can manage any one of these "particular" alcoholic beverages each time you have it in the best way possible.

24. "Sora, can anyone use this program?"

Before starting any weight-loss program particularly if you're diabetic or have high cholesterol it's always important to meet with a doctor or any other licensed health professional. They will help you make an informed decision.

Chapter 12

YOU CAN DO IT!

I decided to end this book with a poem. A poem that supports YOU in finding the success that you deserve with your present weight-loss challenge. The poem is called You Can Do It! You'll find the poem beneath *your* picture.

YOU

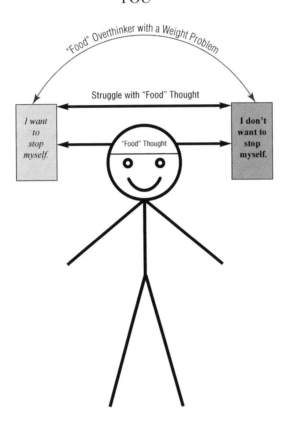

YOU CAN DO IT!

First there's the part of you

that wants to stop!

Then there's the part of you

that doesn't want to stop!

It's your choice to use *your markers* or **"Binge" Foods.**

It's your choice to make friends with food.

It's your choice to know that you can stop yourself.

Success is your choice!

So choose it!

Sora

Sora's Note

You've completed reading this book and I'm really proud of you. I'm proud of the effort that you've made to learn a new way to manage your very own food-thoughts. I'm proud of the effort that you've made to embrace food as your friend and I'm proud that you're choosing to no longer let food torment you.

Be proud of yourself and go for it!

In addition, I would love to be in contact with you through your subscription to my site www.nodieting.net so I can share more thoughts about the wonderful world of no-dieting with you!

Also if you're a member of a Book Club, a Weight Loss Group or a Health Centered or Spiritually Centered Meetup Group and would like to have a Skype *No Diet Event* then just let me know!

Also if you'd like to share your thoughts on the Program with me then you can email me at sora@nodieting.net or write a review on Amazon.

Sora

Program Glossary

Your Self-Stopping Program Terms

l. **"Binge"**-when you switch your thinking from any of your food-thoughts to its matching preselected "Binge" Food so that you know that you can "binge" and stop yourself unlike when diet "bingeing" and feeling out of control.

2. **"Binge" Cold-Drink**-the only cold-drink that you can "binge" on in Program and know that you have stopped yourself.

3. **"Binge" Food**-the only food that you can "binge" on in Program and know that you have stopped yourself.

4. **"Binge" Gum**-the only gum that you can "binge" on in Program and know that you have stopped yourself.

5. **"Binge" Hot-Drink**-the only hot-drink that you can "binge" on in Program and know that you have stopped yourself.

6. **"Binge" Liquids**-your "Binge" Cold-Drink and your "Binge" Hot-Drink are your two Program "binge" liquids.

7. **Bloat**-when you decide to have food that will stuff your stomach on a low caloric intake.

8. **Bloat "Binge"**-when you switch your thinking from your original "bloatable" food thought to your preselected Bloat "Binge" Food so you know that you can stop your bloat "binge" behavior.

9. **Bloat "Binge" Food**-the only type of "bloatable" food that you can "binge" on in Program and know that you have stopped yourself.

10. **Bloat "Eat"**-when as part of The Bloatable's Procedure you decide to "bloat" on a low caloric chewable and use The "Green" Technique to stop yourself.

11. **Bloat "Drunk"**- when as part of The Bloatable's Procedure you decide to "bloat" on a low caloric liquid and use The "Green" Technique to stop yourself.

12. **Bloatables**-any low caloric type of chewable or liquid that you can stuff your stomach on for extreme fullness without having a lot of calories.

13. **"Bloatable" Food Thought**-any time you're thinking about a chewable or a liquid that you purposely want to "bloat" on for a "stuffed" stomach without the calories.

14. **"Bloatable" Food Thought Struggle-**when you're thinking about a bloatable type of chewable or liquid "food" thought and don't know whether you want to stop your "bloatable" food thought and intake or not.

15. **Cold-Drink "Binge"-**when you switch your thinking from your original "cold-drink" thought to your preselected "Binge" Cold-Drink so that you can stop your cold-drink "binge" behavior.

16. **"Cold-Drink" Thought-**when you think about a "cold-drink".

17. **Chewable-**any food or gum that you have to "chew" to digest.

18. **Chewable "Food-Thought" Struggle-**when you're focused to a food or gum thought and you don't know whether you want to stop your food or gum thought or not and therefore stop your chewing behavior or not.

19. **"Chewable" Marker-**the amount of food or gum that you first set aside when using The "Green" Technique that lets you know that you've "eaten" and stopped yourself.

20. **"Cold-Drink" Thought Struggle-**when as part of your struggle with your food-thoughts you don't know whether you're going to stop your "cold-drink" thought and intake or not.

21. **Craving**-a "craving" is a "food" thought. It can be any Inside or Outside "Food-Thought" Caller.

22. **Diet**-a group of rules created by a person or a group of people that more than less tell you what foods to have, when to have them and not to trust your own food-thoughts.

23. **Drink**-when as part of The Stop-Liquid's Procedure you use The "Green" Technique to have the choice to "drink" and stop yourself.

24. **Eat**-when as part of The Stop-Chewable's Procedure you use The "Green" Technique to have the choice to "eat" and stop yourself.

25. **Enough-**the amount that you decide will satisfy you when using The "Green" Technique to either "eat" and stop, "drink" and stop or bloat "eat" and stop.

26. **Food "Binge"**-when you switch your thinking from your original "food" thought to your preselected "Binge" Food so you can stop your food "binge" behavior.

27. **Food "Overbingeing"-**when you see that you're having "too" much of your "Binge" Food and that's what's keeping your weight on.

28. **Food "Overeating"-**when you see that you're Program "eating" too much food with a marker and that's what's keeping your weight on.

29. **"Food" Overthinker-**a person who thinks more about food a day than a person who doesn't and as a result feels feels stuck in a weight problem.

30. **"Food" Thought-**when you think about a "specific" food.

31. **"Food" Thought Struggle-**when as part of your struggle with your food-thoughts you don't know whether you're going to want to stop your "food" thought and your intake or not.

32. **Food-Thought Challenged-**Program says that you don't have the consistent choice to stop visually repeating any "food" thought or any combination of food-thoughts when you decide to, which leaves you thinking more a day about food than a person without a weight problem and therefore feeling stuck in one.

33. **Food-Thoughts-**this term includes all your daily food-thoughts.

34. **Food-Thought Struggle-**the name of the struggle that manages your weight problem and that includes "all" the different types of foods that you think about each day.

35. **Gum "Binge"-**when you decide to switch your thinking from your original "gum" thought to your preselected "Binge" Gum to stop your gum "binge" behavior.

36. **"Gum" Thought-**when you think about a "gum."

37. **"Gum" Thought Struggle**-when as part of your struggle with your food-thoughts you don't know whether you're going to want to stop your "gum" thought and your intake or not.

38. **Hot-Drink "Binge"**-when you decide to switch your thinking from your original "hot-drink" thought to your preselected "Binge" Hot-Drink so you can stop your hot-drink "binge" behavior.

39. **"Hot-Drink" Thought**-when you think about a "hot-drink".

40. **"Hot-Drink" Thought Struggle**-when as part of your struggle with your food-thoughts you don't know whether you're going to want to stop your hot-drink thought and your intake or not.

41. **Inside "Cold-Drink" Caller**-when your body sends you an inner cold-drink/thirst signal and you think about a particular type of cold-drink that will make "that" signal feel better. That feeling better or "match" lets you know that it's the cold-drink that your body is calling for.

42. **Inside "Food" Caller**-when your body sends you an inner "hunger" signal and you think about a particular type of food that will make "that" signal feel better. That feeling better or "match" lets you know that it's the food that your body is calling for.

43. **Inside "Food-Thought" Caller-**any chewable or liquid "food-thought" that you think about as a result of <u>first</u> receiving an inner "hunger" signal or an inner "thirst" signal.

44. **Inside "Gum" Caller-**when your mouth sends you a "mouth/discomfort" signal (to chew) and you think about a particular type of gum that will make that signal feel better. That feeling better or "match" lets you know that that it's the gum that your mouth wants.

45. **Inside "Hot-Drink" Caller-**when your body sends you an inner hot-drink/thirst signal and you think about a particular type of hot-drink that will make "that" signal feel better. That feeling better or "match" lets you know that it's the hot-drink that your body is calling for.

46. **Liquid-**any cold-drink or hot-drink that you have to "drink" to digest.

47. **Liquid "Food-Thought" Struggle-**when you're focused to a cold-drink or a hot-drink thought and you don't know whether you want to stop your cold-drink or hot-drink thought or not and therefore stop your drinking behavior or not.

48. **"Liquid" Marker-**the amount of cold-drink or hot-drink that you remember to leave over when using The "Green" Technique that lets you know that you drank and stopped yourself.

49. **Marker ("Too" Much Marker)**-the amount as part of The "Green" Technique that when set aside either before or after you've respectively eaten, bloat "eaten" or drunk that lets you know that you've chewed or drank and stopped yourself.

50. **Outside "Cold-Drink" Caller**-when you're focused to a cold-drink but received no inner "cold-drink/thirst" signal.

51. **Outside "Food" Caller**-when you're focused to a "food" thought but received no inner "hunger" signal.

52. **Outside "Food-Thought" Caller**-any food or liquid that you think about without having first received an inner "hunger" signal or an inner "thirst" signal.

53. **Outside "Gum" Caller**-when you're focused to a gum thought but your mouth received no inner "need to chew/discomfort" signal.

54. **Outside "Hot-Drink" Caller**-when you're focused to a hot-drink but received no inner "hot-drink/thirst" signal.

55. **"Overbinge"**-when you observe that you're having "too" much of your "Binge" Food to comfortably reach your non-dieted weight loss goal.

56. **"Overeat"**-when you use The "Green" Technique to eat but feel that you've had "too" much.

57. **Program "binge"**-Program "bingeing" is when you "binged" on one of your five preselected "Binge" Foods which lets you know that you have stopped your respective "binge" behavior.

58. **Program "eat"**-Program "eating" is when you use The "Green" Technique with a "chewable" marker, know that you've had "enough" and know that you've had the choice to eat and stop yourself.

59. **Program "drink"**-Program "drinking" is when you use The "Green" Technique with a "liquid" marker, know that you've had "enough" and know that you've had the choice to drink and stop yourself.

60. **Sora's Weight-Loss "Management" Program**-the name of the program which lets you manage your "own" food-thoughts without dieting. The Program includes three self-stopping food-thought "management" procedures and three additional special weight-loss "management" strategies.

61. **Struggle with "Food" Thought**-means the "same" as "food" thought struggle.

62. **The Bloatable's Procedure-**is the third self-stopping food-thought "management" procedure in Sora's Weight-Loss "Management" Program. It lets you decrease your weight-loss "management" time through the choice of a low caloric stuffed stomach.

63. **The Bloatable's Procedure Demo Form-**the format that the book uses to teach you how to use The Bloatable's Procedure.

64. **The "Boredom" Technique-**one of the three special weight-loss "management" strategies which tells you to "food" binge to excess (and not food "overeat" with a marker) so that food "bingeing" boredom sets in sooner than later for a non-dieted weight-loss choice.

65. **The Daily Program Form-**the name of the form that you can use to record your daily self-stopped, Program choices.

66. **The "4" Technique-**one of the three special weight-loss "management" strategies which encourages you not to food "overeat" or not to food "overbinge" but instead to choose to have either your 4 lower caloric foods with a marker or your 4 lower caloric "Binge" foods without a marker.

67. **The "Green" Technique-**is the name of one of the techniques in each of The Program's 3 self-stopping food-thought "management" procedures. It gives you the choice to eat and stop, drink and stop or bloat and stop by using a "Too" Much Marker.

68. **The "Minimizer" Technique-**one of the three special weight-loss "management" strategies that tells you to cut back whether you're food "overeating" with a marker or food "overbingeing".

69. **The "Red" Technique-**the name of one the techniques in each of The Program's 3 self-stopping food-thought "management" procedures. It always gives you the choice to "binge" and know that you have stopped yourself.

70. **The Stop-Chewable's Procedure-**is the first self-stopping, food-thought "management" procedure in Sora's Weight-Loss "Management" Program. The procedure lets you have any food or gum that you want and be able to stop yourself whether as part of your Chewable "Food-Thought" Struggle you either want to chew and stop yourself or not.

71. **The Stop-Chewable's Procedure Demo Form-**the format that the book uses to teach you how to use The Stop-Chewable's Procedure.

72. **The Stop-Liquid's Procedure-**is the second self-stopping, food-thought "management" procedure in Sora's Weight-Loss "Management" Program. The procedure lets you have any cold-drink or hot-drink that you want and be able to stop yourself whether as part of your Liquid "Food-Thought" Struggle you either want to drink and stop yourself or not.

73. **The Stop-Liquid's Procedure Demo Form**-the format that the book uses to teach you how to use The Stop-Liquid's Procedure.

74. **"Too" Much Marker (Marker)**-the amount as part of The "Green" Technique that when set aside either before or after you've respectively eaten, bloat "eaten" or drunk that lets you know that you've chewed or drunk and stopped yourself.

Appendix

If you're reading the Kindle version of this book then go to www.nodieting.net and you'll find your link to the book's appendix. Your code for your download is the first word in Chapter 3.

Helpful Hints When Using "Chewable" Markers

Here are some helpful hints when you've decided that you want to eat and stop yourself and you need to first set aside a "chewable" marker.

Example #1-I want the whole bag of Cheese Bits.

If you decide that you want the whole bag of Cheese Bits, then you can have it but you still have to leave a marker.

In this case, just scrape off a little bit from one of your Cheese Bits and leave it under your fingernail.

Then eat the amount that you decided was enough but never the amount under your fingernail.

This will let you know that you have eaten and stopped yourself.

This under the fingernail rule applies anytime you want to eat all the food in the package and want the choice to stop yourself.

You must know where your marker is.

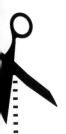

Example #2-Food from a bag or box

You have to use the same "under your fingernail" rule when you're having food from a "larger" type of bag or box and don't want the whole thing.

So for example, let's say that you want Oreos and you've decided that you want to eat and stop yourself.

You'll get your large box of Oreos and let's say for teaching purposes that you want 5.

You'll take out the 5 Oreos that you want and then put the rest away.

However, before you can eat the 5 Oreos you have to scrape off a marker from one of your Oreos and leave it under your fingernail.

This will let you know that you can eat your 5 Oreos and stop yourself.

Now if you decide that you want more Oreos, from that "same" box, then you have to follow that "same" procedure again.

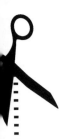

Example #3-Several Foods on a Plate

When you have several foods on your plate such as chicken, broccoli and a potato and you know that you want to eat and stop yourself then you're going to have to set aside a marker for each of those foods.

You'll decide how much of the chicken is enough (and how much is "too" much), how much of the broccoli is enough (and how much is "too" much) and how much of the potato is enough and how much is "too" much.

Then you're going to want to physically separate all 3 of your food markers on the plate from the amounts that you decided were enough.

That's when you need to think about your plate as a clock and pick a favorite time such as 6:00 P.M. found at the bottom of your plate.

Then put all your markers at 6:00 P.M. so that when you're eating the amounts that you decided were enough, your markers are safe and separate.

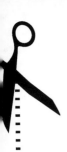

A Helpful Hint When Using a "Liquid" Marker

Here is a helpful hint when you've decided that you want to drink and stop yourself and you need to leave over a "liquid" marker.

Helpful Hint:

If you're pouring juice or any liquid from a bottle or a container then you have to pour in more than enough to know that you'll be able to "see" your left over marker.

It's not enough to think that your marker is left in the bottle or the container from which you took the liquid.

That's because you have to "see" your "liquid" marker at the bottom of your glass to know that you have truly stopped yourself.

My 5 "Binge" Foods Chart

My "Binge" Food is_____.

My "Binge" Gum is_____.

My "Binge" Cold-Drink is_____.

My "Binge" Hot-Drink is_____.

My Bloat "Binge" Food is_____.

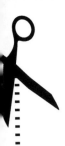

Program Recording Instructions

On the next page you'll find a copy of your Daily Program Form. Cut this page out and make as many copies as you might need.

Let's go over the way that you can record your self-stopping food choices to "*see*" how you're doing.

Anytime you Program "eat" food or gum and use a "Too" Much Marker to stop yourself then record your self-stopped "eating" experience in the first column called Program "eat" ("Too" Much Marker").

Anytime you Program "drink" a cold-drink or hot-drink and use a "Too" Much Marker to stop yourself then record your self-stopped "drinking" experience in the second column called Program "drink" ("Too" Much Marker).

Then, anytime you Program "binge" on any of your 5 "Binge" Foods (to stop yourself), then record your self-stopped "bingeing" experience in the third column called Program "Binge" (5 "Binge" Foods).

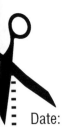

The Daily Program Form

Date: Weight:

Sora's Weight-Loss "Management" Program		
Program "eat" ("Too" Much Marker)	*Program "drink"* ("Too" Much Marker)	**Program "binge"** (5 "Binge" Foods)
Calories:	Calories:	Calories:

Today's Caloric Intake:

The Stop-Chewable's Procedure

1. Before you can have the food or gum that you're thinking about, you have to ask yourself the question:

"Do I want to stop myself or not?"

2. Then you have to wait for your answer to arrive.

3. Once your answer has arrived then you'll know which of The Procedure's two self-stopping techniques you're going to have to use.

Answer: "I want to stop myself."	**Answer: "I don't want to stop myself."**
Use: The "Green" Technique	**Use: The "Red" Technique**

1. Get The Inside or Outside "Food" or "Gum" Caller that you want.	**1. You have to immediately switch your thinking from your original food or gum thought to your preselected "Binge" Food or preselected "Binge" Gum to stop your original food or gum thought.**
2. Ask yourself: "How much is enough and how much is "too" much?"	
3. Set aside the amount which was "too" much.	
4. Eat the amount that you decided was enough.	**2. Then get your preselected "Binge" Food or your preselected "Binge" Gum.**
5. Never eat your "Too" Much Marker.	

This will let you know that you have stopped either your food or gum "eating" behavior.

3. Then ask yourself: How much is a comfortable amount to "binge" on?

4. Then "binge" on that "comfortable" amount.

5. "Binge" on that "comfortable" amount without having to first set aside a "Too" Much Marker.
*This will let you know that you have stopped your food "binge" behavior or your gum "binge" behavior.

The Stop-Liquid's Procedure

1. Before you can have the cold-drink or hot-drink that you're thinking about, you have to ask yourself the question:

"Do I want to stop myself or not?"

2. Then you have to wait for your answer to arrive.

3. Once your answer has arrived then you'll know which of The Procedure's two self-stopping techniques you're going to have to use.

Answer: "I want to stop myself."

Use: The "Green" Technique

Answer: "I don't want to stop myself."

Use: The "Red" Technique

1. Get The Inside or Outside "Cold-Drink" or "Hot-Drink" Caller that you want.

2. Ask yourself: "How much is enough and how much is "too" much?"

3. Have the amount that you decided was enough.

4. Remember to leave over the amount that you decided was "too" much.

5. Then glance at, or swish or shake the amount that you left over, your "Too"

1. You have to immediately switch your thinking from your original cold-drink or hot-drink thought to your preselected "Binge" Cold-Drink or your preselected "Binge" Hot-Drink to stop your original cold-drink or hot-drink thought.

2. Then get your preselected "Binge" Cold-Drink or your preselected "Binge" Hot-Drink.

Much Marker.

* That will let you know that you have stopped either your cold-drink or hot-drink "drinking" behavior.

3. Then ask yourself, "How much is comfortable amount to "binge" on?

4. Then "binge" on that "comfortable" amount.

5. "Binge on that "comfortable" amount without having to remember to leave over a "Too" Much Marker.

*This will let you know that you have stopped your cold-drink "binge" behavior or your hot-drink "binge" behavior.

The Bloatable's Procedure

1. You decide not to have the higher caloric food that you're thinking about but you decide to "bloat" on a lower caloric food instead.

2. Once you switch your thinking to your lower caloric food thought then you have to ask yourself the question:

"Do I want to stop myself or not?"

3. Then you have to wait for your answer to arrive.

Answer: "I want to stop myself."	**Answer: "I don't want to stop myself."**
Use: The "Green" Technique	**Use: The "Red" Technique**

1. Get the "chewable" or "liquid" bloatable that you're thinking of.

1. You have to immediately switch thinking from your original chewable or liquid "bloat" food to your preselected Bloat "Binge" Food to stop your original "bloatable" food thought.

2. Ask yourself, "how much is enough to "bloat" on to stuff my stomach and how much is "too" much?"

3. Then "bloat" on the amount that you decided was enough and don't have your "Too" Much Marker.

2. Then get your Bloat "Binge" Food.

3. Then ask yourself, "how much is a "comfortable" amount to bloat

*If your bloatable is a chewable then you'll set aside your "Too" Much Marker before

you "bloat". If your bloatable is a liquid then you'll remember to leave some over after you've had your enough amount.

****This will let you know that you have either bloat "eaten" or bloat "drunk" and stopped yourself.*

"binge" on?

4. Then bloat "binge" on that "comfortable" amount.

5. Bloat "binge" on that "comfortable" amount without having to first set aside or leave over a "Too" Much Marker.

*This will let you know that you have bloat "binged" and stopped yourself.

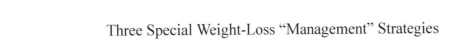

Three Special Weight-Loss "Management" Strategies

The "Minimizer" Technique

With: Food Callers

With "Binge" Foods

Work on cutting back.

Work on cutting back.

The "4" Technique

With: Food Callers

Train yourself not to food

"overeat" with a marker but

to otherwise have gum, a cold-drink,

a hot-drink or a bloatable with a

marker instead.

With: "Binge" Foods

Train yourself not to food

"overbinge" but to otherwise

have your "Binge" Gum, your

"Binge" Cold-Drink, your "Binge

"Hot-Drink" or your Bloat

"Binge" Food instead.

The "Boredom" Technique

(Use The "Boredom" Technique if you've tried

The "Minimizer" Technique and tried The "4" Technique

and you're still struggling to reach your forever thin and

healthy goal).

With: Food Callers

1. Train yourself to have your

   "Binge" Food instead of food

   "overeating" with a marker.

2. Training yourself to food

   "overbinge" instead of

   food "overeat" with a marker

   will make your extra "Binge" Food

   calories more boring in a shorter

   amount of time because of their

   "sameness".

3. That will make it easier for you

   to cut back your food "overbingeing"

   behavior while continuing not to

   food "overeat" with a marker.

With: "Binge" Foods

1. Train yourself to continue to

   food "overbinge" without

   food "overeating" with a

   marker.

2. Continued food "overbingeing"

   will become so boring that you'll

   want to cut back.

3. You'll be able to cut back all the

   while remembering not to

   food "overeat" with a marker.

EASY TO USE PROGRAM FORM

Do I want to stop myself or not?

Yes   No

How much is enough?   Can't have the food!

marker   "Binge" Food

*Always have your "Binge" Food
at hand.

About Sora

Sora Vernikoff, writer, educator and Program developer has worked with hundreds of people who share her vision of life after dieting. Sora lives in Manhattan and loves to go to the theatre and travel. Sora has taught her Program to her private clients, at The Learning Annex and at the office of a leading New York endocrinologist. She has also spoken at Lennox Hill Hospital, and has been on radio and on national television.

Sora is available for presentations, seminars as well as individual and group coaching!

Contact:

Sora@nodieting.net
www.nodieting.net

Index

Made in the USA
Columbia, SC
27 July 2017